Disclaimer

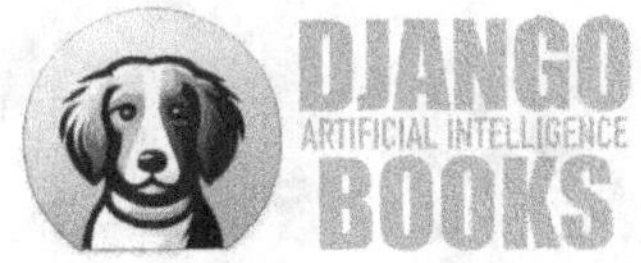

Introduction

Welcome, dear reader, to an odyssey most extraordinary, where silicon synapses meet human pulses, crafting a saga where algorithms not only predict but participate in the pantheon of healthcare. Imagine a world where your watch whispers secrets of your heart's desires —nay, its needs—straight into the ears of digital deities designed to guard and enhance your corporeal vessel. Here, we explore the vast vaults of virtuality where artificial intelligence serves as both shield and sword against the onslaught of ailments and the decay of time.

Our journey, akin to a magnificent symphony, commences with the overture of understanding—what is this beast named AI? As you delve deeper, each chapter unfurls like a lotus of knowledge, petals drenched in the profound elixir of insight, each droplet a revelation. From wearable wonders that monitor your midnight murmurs to bespoke nutritional advice dispensed by your digital dietitian, we traverse a landscape lush with innovation.

Picture this: a digital therapist who doesn't just nod but knows, truly comprehends the labyrinthine pathways of

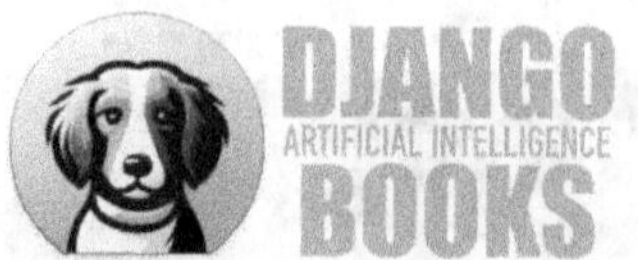

Table of Contents

(Click to Quick-Jump to Chapters)

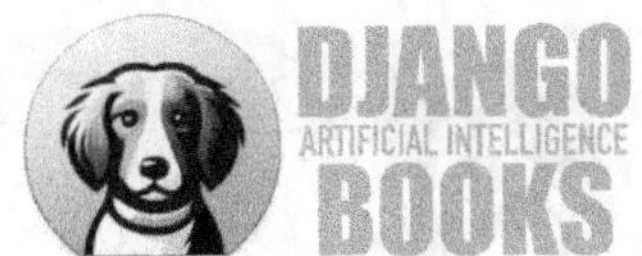

Copyright

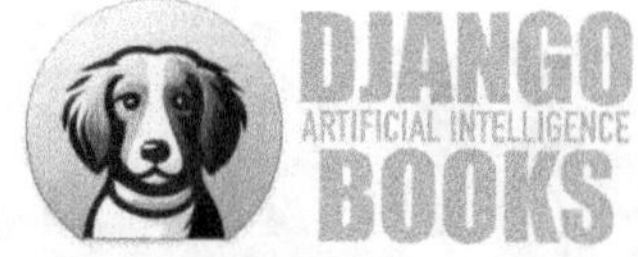

your mind, offering solace and solutions without ever interrupting. Or envision a scenario where your very genetic fabric is deciphered by algorithms more adept than any human hand, tailoring treatments as personally as a tailor from Savile Row would craft your suit. These are not mere fantasies from a futurist's fever dream but palpable realities, ready to be grasped with eager hands.

Yet, as we gallivant gleefully through this garden of technological delights, let us not overlook the thorns among the roses. Ethical enigmas abound, privacy predicaments poke at every turn, and the specter of inequality looms like a storm cloud over Eden. How do we navigate this brave new world with wisdom, ensuring that these potent powers are wielded for wellness and not woe?

So buckle up, adjust your reading spectacles, and prepare your intellect for a feast. You are not merely reading a tome; you are stepping onto a carousel of upgrades celebration, where each turn brings new vistas of possibility. This book is not only your guide but also your gateway to an augmented future where health is not just managed but mastered. Let the pages turn, let the algorithms churn, and let us embark on this remarkable

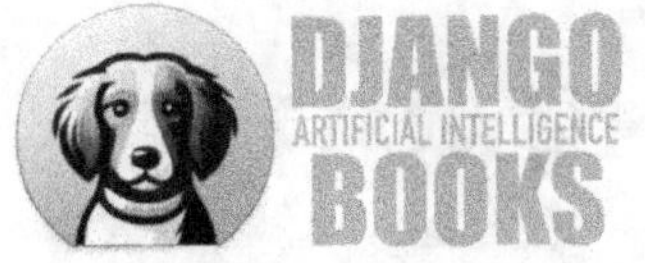

adventure, for AI-enhanced health—improved by the very essence of ingenuity—is a tale worth telling.

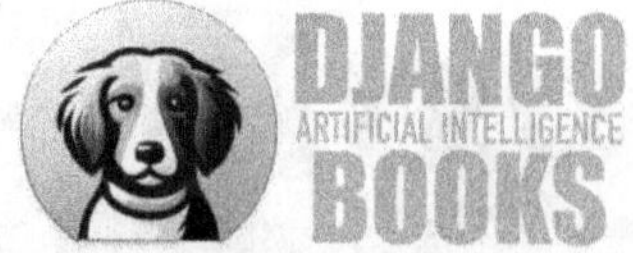

Chapter 1: Deciphering the Digital Doctorate, Understanding AI's Role in Health

Embarking upon an odyssey through the annals of medicinal marvels, one encounters the genesis of artificial intelligence in healthcare—a narrative not merely of technological triumph but of an exquisite intertwining of silicon with stethoscopes. This inaugural exploration elucidates the profound transformation from rudimentary record-keeping to a sophisticated symphony of data-driven diagnostics, a journey where erstwhile fantasies of robotic assistance have crystallized into the quotidian realities of clinical practice.

In the hallowed halls of history, one discerns that the concept of artificial intelligence—a phantasmagoric notion once confined to the realms of science fiction—began its flirtation with medicine as early as the mid-20th century. Initial forays were tentative, marked by machines of modest means, tasked with the mere mimicry of human cognition.

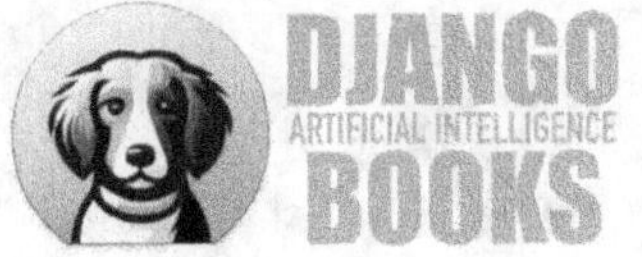

However, as the digital age dawned, these mechanical minds evolved from simple calculators to profound prognosticators, capable of dissecting vast volumes of data with voracious velocity and viper-like precision.

Consider the early systems developed to diagnose illnesses, primitive yet prescient heralds of the AI revolution. These systems, though initially as cumbersome as a convocation of clumsy clerics, gradually gained the grace of gazelles, galloping through genetic information and imaging data to discern and detail the diabolical details of diseases. The transformation was not instantaneous but an iterative infusion of intellect into inanimate objects, driven by the dual desires of accuracy and efficiency.

Advancing further into this technological tapestry, one must appreciate the role of algorithms in augmenting the acuity of assessments. These algorithmic architects, wielding their computational chisels, sculpt the raw marble of medical data into the discernible figures of diagnostic relevance. The sagacity of such systems becomes apparent in their capacity to capture nuances in data that elude even the eagle eyes of experienced examiners, thus heralding an era where predictive prowess is paramount.

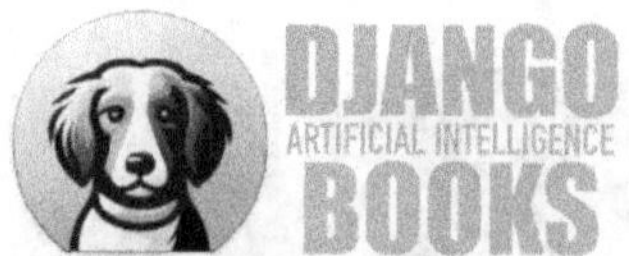

The labyrinthine linkage between computational capabilities and clinical outcomes becomes even more labyrinthine when considering the international contributions to this corpus of knowledge. From the silicon valleys of the United States to the tech-savvy terrains of Taiwan, a confluence of global genius has propelled the proliferation of AI in healthcare, making it a veritable vessel of international innovation. Each geographic contribution layers additional complexity and nuance, enriching the entire enterprise with a diverse array of analytical angles.

Moreover, the ethical implications inherent in integrating artificial intelligence into the intimate intricacies of individual health care are neither trivial nor tepid. As these digital doctors delve deeper into the domains traditionally dominated by human decision-makers, questions quiver in the quagmire about the moral matrices within which these machines must operate. The privacy of patient data, the potential for programming prejudice, and the palpable fear of dehumanizing decisions are but a few of the formidable challenges that frolic fiendishly at the forefront of this fascinating field.

Thus, as we stand at the precipice of this paradigmatic shift in healthcare, one cannot help but marvel at the

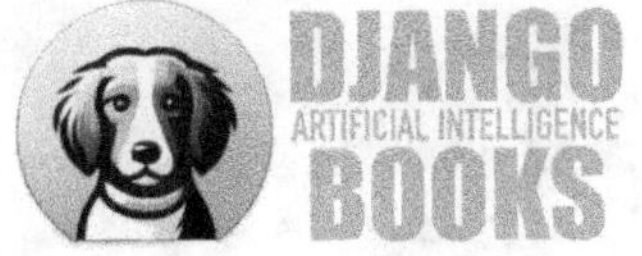

metamorphosis mediated by these magnificent mechanical minds. The journey from the mechanical to the medical, from data points to diagnoses, encapsulates an epoch characterized by both colossal challenges and staggering strides. Herein lies not just a tale of technology but a profound parable of progress, promise, and the perpetual pursuit of perfection in the protection and preservation of human health. As we turn each page of this ongoing saga, let us tread thoughtfully, tempering our technological triumphs with a touch of timeless humanity.

In the sanctum of scientific sophistication, one encounters a veritable vista of complexities when attempting to delineate the multifarious dimensions of Artificial Intelligence, particularly its resplendent roles and rigorous responsibilities within the realm of healthcare. Our discourse shall delve into the intricacies of this enigmatic entity, unwinding its coiled complexities with the precision of a virtuoso violinist engaged in a capricious cadenza.

As we traverse the intricate inner workings of AI, it becomes palpably apparent that we are not merely observing a series of sterile silicon operations, but rather a grandiose theatrical production. Here, algorithms assume the roles of protagonists, their every calculation and

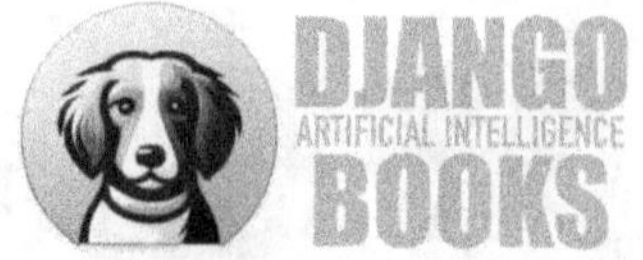

decision choreographed like a ballet in binary. These algorithmic actors, donning the costumes of code, perform on the grand stage of medical data, their performances meticulously directed by the maestros of machine learning to foster feats of diagnostic and therapeutic dexterity.

Venturing into the anatomy of these algorithms, we explore the layers of learning that constitute their core. At the embryonic stage, these algorithms are akin to naive novices, empty canvases eager to be etched with the empirical essences of experiential data. Through a pedagogical process known as 'training', these fledgling formulas feast on vast volumes of variegated data, from radiographic revelations to pathological pronouncements. It is within this crucible of computation that the algorithms evolve from mere data devourers to sagacious savants, capable of unveiling veiled verities within the health histories they dissect.

Applications of these learned logicians span a spectacular spectrum, from the quotidian to the quixotic. On one hand, we witness the workaday wizardry of wearable wellness monitors, these diligent devices continuously collecting corporeal clues and dispatching data-driven health harbingers directly to one's digital

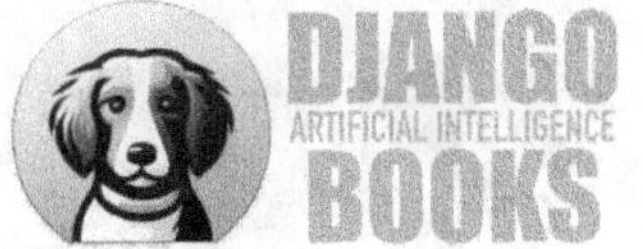

doorstep. On the other hand, one marvels at the meticulous machinations of robotic surgical systems, where AI assumes an almost artisanal agency, its precise incisions guided by the gentle governance of algorithmic insight. These robotic virtuosos perform with such finesse that even the steadiest of human hands might yield to the yoke of envy.

However, the application of AI in healthcare is not without its moments of melodrama and missteps. Instances abound where algorithms, in their zealous zest for zeroing in on zoonotic zeniths, have occasionally concocted conclusions that could charitably be described as comically confounding. Picture, if you will, a scenario where an AI, in its infinite inferential ingenuity, diagnoses a hiccup as harbinger of some horrendous, yet wholly hypothetical health hazard. Such sallies into the surreal serve as salient reminders of the necessity for nuanced navigation of these neural networks, ensuring that their counsel remains cogent and their deductions, despite occasional detours into the domain of the delirious, generally guide us towards greater good.

In summation, while the detailed delineation of AI's anatomy reveals a structure both sublime and sometimes

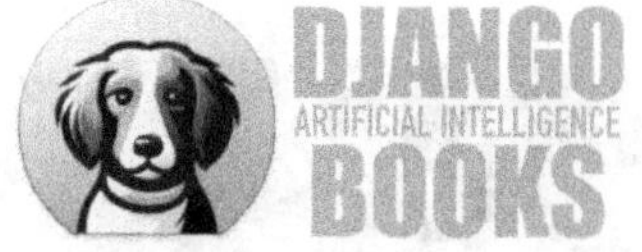

susceptible to the slings and arrows of outrageous outputs, the overarching odyssey of these algorithmic auteurs is one marked by a majestic melding of machine-based meticulousness and medical mastery. As this narrative unfurls, swathed in the swaddling of sophisticated science and speckled with the spice of serendipitous slips, one cannot help but anticipate the next act in this audacious adventure, where algorithms not only inform but transform the very tapestry of therapeutic tradition.

In an epoch where oracles are not perched atop Delphic mounts but are rather ensconced within the enigmatic embrace of silicon circuits, the realm of predictive health analytics emerges as a paragon of prophetic precision. Herein, the sagacity of algorithms transcends mere mortal measure, imbuing data with the divinatory powers to preemptively pronounce the potentials of pathological perturbations.

Delving deeper into this digital Delphi, one encounters the algorithms – those meticulous maestros of mathematical musing – that deftly derive, from the dense and often disorderly detritus of data, predictions with a precision that would make Pythia herself pale in prophetic envy. These algorithmic augurs, laboring in the labyrinthine

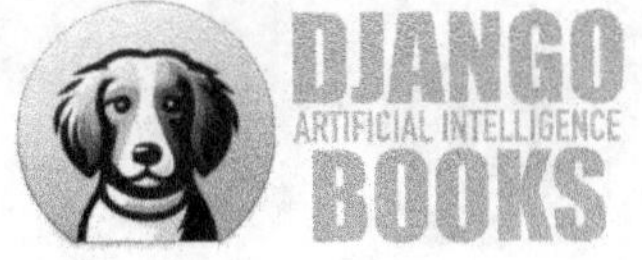

limbo between raw data and refined deduction, weave the wondrous web of what might, with high probability, occur in the corpus humanum, given the ghostly guidance of gigabytes gone by.

Consider the colossal capability of these computational clairvoyants to foresee the foibles of the flesh before they manifest into maladies. A mere murmur in the metabolic makeup, a subtle shift in synaptic sequences, or an innocuous anomaly in immunological indices might not catch the clinician's eye. Yet, to these predictive prodigies, such signs are as stark as a supernova in a starless sky. Armed with the arcane arts of artificial neural networks, support vector machines, and random forests (to name but a few of their number), these algorithms analyze and anticipate, offering omens of oncoming ailments with an alacrity that belies the complexity of their calculations.

One must also marvel at the jocular juxtaposition of AI's predictive prowess in its nascent stage, where its prognostications could sometimes seem as if divined by a dice roll – a digital drollery of diagnostics. For instance, envision an early algorithmic attempt to predict flu trends, which, mistaking the seasonal spike in searches for

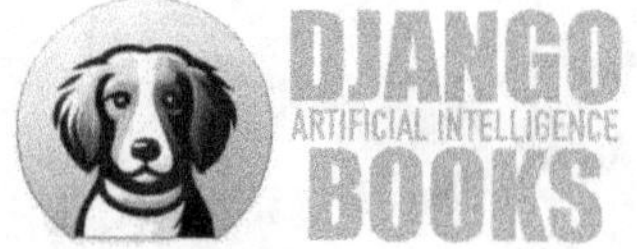

chicken soup recipes as an indicator of a forthcoming flu epidemic, might have ludicrously led to a run on broth rather than influenza vaccinations. These hiccups, while highlighting the heuristic hurdles of early analytics, also underscore the undulating journey from whimsical guesses to weighted guidance.

Yet, it is not solely in the solitary soothsaying where these predictive protocols ply their potent trade. Their integration into the interstices of interactive health management systems where patients and providers alike can ponder upon the portended possibilities and prepare accordingly, ushers a new era of engaged, enlightened, and perhaps even emancipated health experiences. Such systems do not merely serve as passive portals of prophetic pronouncements but as dynamic dialogues where human and machine, in concert, contemplate and counteract the creeping shadows of sickness.

Furthermore, the beneficence of these predictive paradigms blooms brilliantly in their capacity to equalize the echelons of healthcare accessibility. With predictive analytics, remote regions bereft of bountiful medical expertise can still benefit from the bounty of big data's prognostic power, thus democratizing the diagnostics and

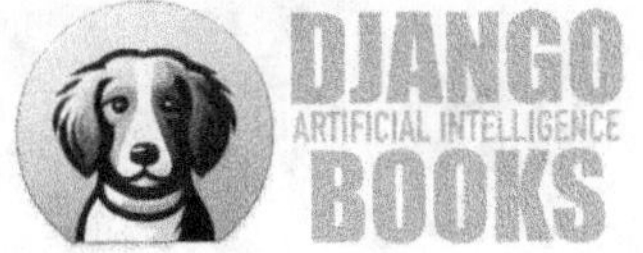

deftly distributing the dividends of digital health developments.

In sum, the prophetic precision of predictive health analytics stands as a testament to the triumphant transmutation of terabytes into tenable, tangible, and timely health tenets. As we wade deeper into this wondrous wellspring of wisdom, where whimsy meets weighty forewarning, the horizons of health care expand exponentially, ensuring that each individual not only anticipates the advent of ailments but also arms themselves against the arcane assaults of the unforeseen. Thus, this narrative unfolds, not merely as a chronicle of computational conquests but as a vibrant vignette of visionary vigor, volleying forth into the vast vistas of vitality.

In the grand tapestry of technological triumphs, the interweaving of artificial intelligence within the sanctum of medicine is not without its prickly ethical enigmas and confounding confidentiality conundrums. As these digital denizens delve into the deepest recesses of our biological being, they stir a tempest of dilemmas that rattle the very cage of contemporary medical ethics, prompting a profound pondering over privacy, propriety, and the precarious balance between beneficence and intrusion.

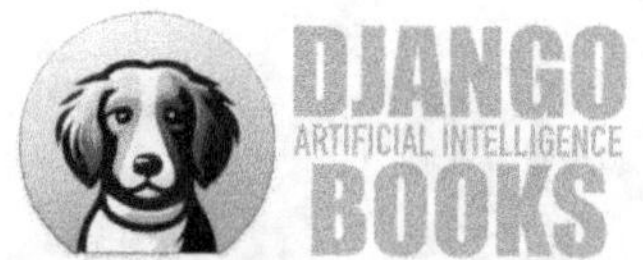

Embark, if you will, on an intellectual jaunt through the jungles of judgment where AI, the audacious interloper, challenges the sacrosanctity of secrets once whispered in the hallowed confidentiality of a doctor's chambers. The question quivers in the quagmire: how does one ensure that these algorithmic arbiters of health adhere to the Hippocratic oath, particularly in their handling of the hallowed hieroglyphs of health data? This conundrum casts a colossal shadow over the utilitarian utopia promised by personalized medicine.

One might chortle at the irony of an AI, sophisticated beyond the ken of most mortals, yet potentially as porous in privacy as a sieve in a storm. Imagine, a scenario where sensitive health data, rather than being securely siloed, becomes an inadvertent broadcast in a breach most bizarre, leading to a ludicrous lineup of unsolicited advertisements for ailments unannounced. The slapstick scenario, while exaggerated, underscores the grave gambit of guarding our most guarded guises against the gargantuan appetite of data-driven diagnostics.

Yet, the ethical entanglements extend beyond the mere mechanics of data discretion. Consider the conundrum of decision-making dominance: should the

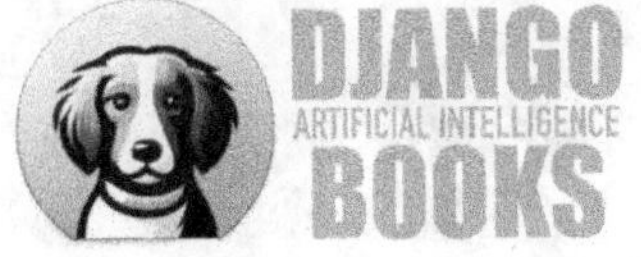

silicon savant serve as mere consultant, or could it conceivably commandeer the clinical decisions, relegating the human healer to a handmaiden of hardware? This scenario, rife with the risible notion of a doctor deferring to the diagnostic decrees of a digital deity, ignites a fiery debate among the erudite echelons of medical ethicists. One muses on the absurdity of a medical maestro, years in training, turning to a tablet for therapeutic tutelage as if seeking the wisdom of an oracle.

Moreover, delve deeper into the ethical quagmire with the consideration of algorithmic autonomy. The potential for an AI to develop diagnostic biases based on skewed datasets is not merely a theoretical thicket but a practical pitfall. The risk juts out like a sore thumb when one envisions an AI, trained in the verdant valleys of one continent, vainly venturing verdicts on the varied vicissitudes of a vastly different demographic, with the blithe blundering of a bull in a china shop.

In the realm of resolutions, the dialogue delves into the development of robust regulatory frameworks that aim to tame the tempestuous tides of technology. The establishment of stringent standards and the vigilant vetting of AI applications in health care could serve as bulwarks

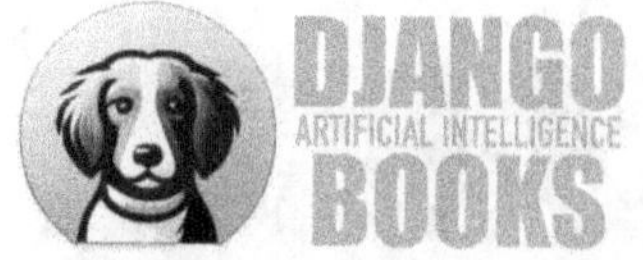

against the breaches of both ethics and encryption. The prospect of international coalitions crafting cohesive codes of conduct for computational care conjures images of digital diplomats, negotiating the nuances of neural networks, in a bid to build a bastion of both beneficence and confidentiality.

Thus, as we wade through the weighty waters of ethical exploration, the journey through these conundrums is neither trivial nor tepid. It is a vibrant voyage that vaults beyond the veneer of technological triumphs to touch the tender tissue of human trust and moral moorings. Each step in this saga, steeped in both seriousness and a sprinkle of satire, adds a valuable veneer to the voluminous discourse on the virtuous deployment of AI in the venerable vocation of medicine.

As we gallantly galavant into the grandiloquent garden of empirical elucidation, a careful consideration of AI's efficacy in healthcare emerges not merely as an exercise in intellectual indulgence but as a profound pilgrimage to the pinnacles of peer-reviewed prudence. This exploration, draped in the dense drapery of data and dotted with the delightful dollops of discovery, delves deep into the dominions where artificial intelligence has been

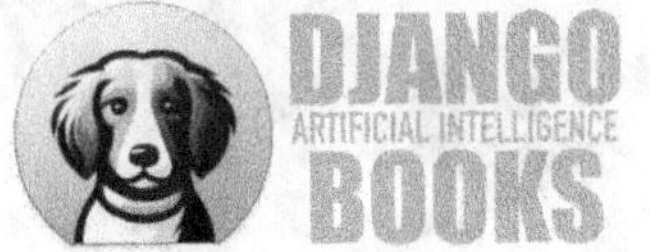

meticulously measured against the milestones of medical mastery.

Embarking on this expedition, one is immediately struck by the lusciously labyrinthine literature that lauds the laurels of AI's accomplishments in various vicinities of the vast healthcare vista. The spectacle unfolds somewhat akin to a high-stakes horse race, where every algorithmic avatar is a thoroughbred thundering through the theoretical tracks, cheered on by clusters of clinicians and statisticians brandishing their betting slips of bibliographies.

A first stop in this fantastical fairground is the radiology rodeo, where AI, equipped with the ethereal eagle-eye, excels at elucidating the enigmas ensconced within esoteric echograms and enigmatic X-rays. Imagine, if you will, the scenario of AI outperforming even the most sagacious of seasoned radiologists, detecting derelictions in the depths of diagnostic images with a deftness that dances delicately on the line between dazzling and downright supernatural. Studies systematically show that in identifying idiosyncrasies like insidious intracranial bleeds or the subtle shadows of pulmonary pathologies, these digital detectives deploy a precision that practically

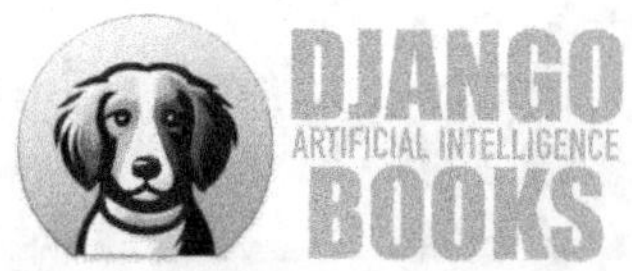

prognosticates the pending applause from astounded audiences.

Progressing past the pictorial prowess of AI, we wade into the waters of wearable wellness gadgets. These devices, donned daily by the diligent and the debonair alike, collect copious counts of cardiovascular and corporeal cues. Here, the AI acts as an analytical alchemist, transmuting the torrential tides of terabytes into tangible, tractable tips that teeter tantalizingly on the brink of bespoke behavioral advice. One's smartwatch might be scolding softly for a skipped session at the gym or a surreptitiously snacked slice of cake, yet the underlying utility underscores a serious stride towards sustaining superb health standards.

Moreover, the tale twists tantalizingly as one treads towards the trials and tribulations of treatment plans tailored through AI. In the oncological opera, algorithms orchestrate an opus of optimized, personalized protocols, outpacing the old, one-size-fits-all approach with an agility akin to a virtuoso violinist deftly delivering a dazzlingly difficult Paganini caprice. Peer-reviewed papers pompously proclaim the prowess of these protocols, presenting a

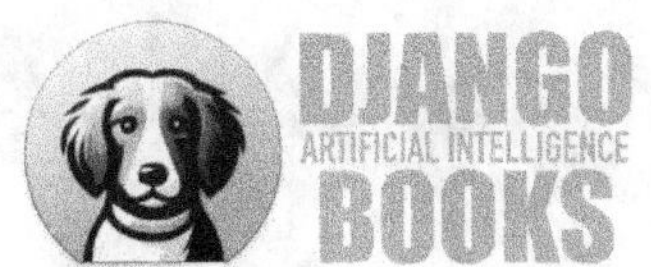

parade of patients potentially spared the peregrination through the more perilous pathways of pharmacotherapy.

Yet, not all is mirth and merriment in the meticulous measuring of these machinations. Skeptics, armed with a healthy heaping of hesitance, hoist hefty inquiries into the reproducibility and robustness of results, igniting incendiary debates in illustrious institutions. The scene could be compared to a grand, gastronomical gathering where each critique of AI's efficacy is a spicy, sizzling steak served searing hot, challenging the palates and perceptions of partaking patrons.

In summation, evaluating the efficacy of AI in healthcare demands a discerning dive into a deluge of data, a feat that is as foreboding as it is fundamentally fascinating. Through this laborious, yet lighthearted journey into the jubilant jungle of peer-reviewed revelations, one is left not merely educated but armed with the assurance that the future of healthcare, held in the hearty hands of high-tech, heralds a horizon replete with hope, and the highest standards of health.

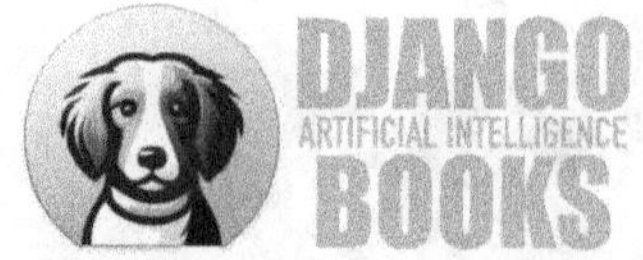

Chapter 2: Transformative Tech, AI Devices That Monitor and Manage Health

Venture now, if you dare, into the vivacious vortex of variable velocity where wearables and sensorial wonders form a pantheon of technological prodigies, each more eager than the last to whisper the arcane secrets of your corporeal constitution directly into the digital ether. This grandiloquent gala of gadgets galore is not merely an assortment of devices; it represents an armada of AI-enhanced artifacts, each armed to the teeth with an arsenal of sensors, poised to plunder the depths of your physiological phenomena with piratical precision.

Picture, in your mind's recesses, the quintessential smartwatch, an unassuming sentinel on your wrist, ever vigilant. Far from being a simple timekeeper, this device is imbued with the intelligence of a miniature maestro, conducting a continuous symphony of data collection. Heart rate, sleep patterns, steps taken, and even the

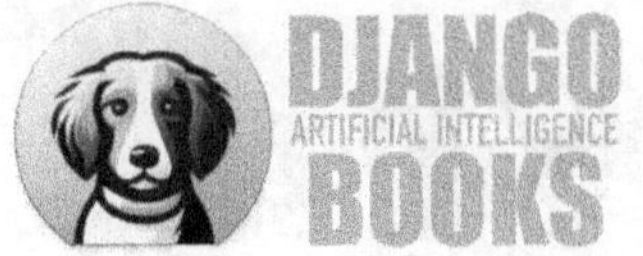

nuances of your nocturnal natterings are meticulously monitored, measured, and marshaled into meaningful insights about your health. The absurdity that a device strapped snugly against your skin could potentially know more about your physical well-being than you do yourself, flirts perilously with the preposterous!

Advancing deeper into the sensorial sanctum, one encounters the esoteric echelons of embedded health trackers, ingeniously integrated into the very fabric of daily life. Clothing—yes, clothing—endowed with the cunning to count calories, compute cardiovascular coherence, and even catch early symptoms of corporeal crises, masquerades as mere mundane attire. Imagine your socks sagely advising you to sit due to an impending spike in blood pressure, or your shirt subtly suggesting a salubrious stretch—such sartorial advisors transform the very tapestry of textile technology.

Let us not bypass the bizarre ballet of the bathroom scales, those unsung urchins of the utility room, now reimagined as oracles of obesity and overseers of osteal density. With a step upon their unassuming platforms, they unleash their latent lore of your bodily burden, offering omens of weighty matters through a cold, calculating gaze

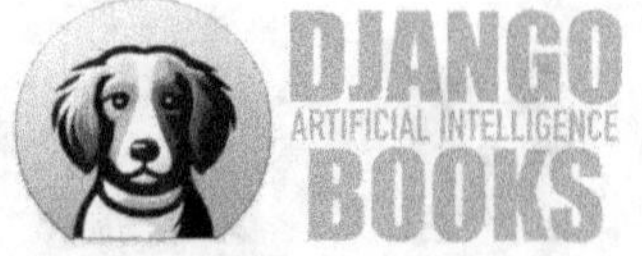

upon your gravitational pull. The jocular juxtaposition of a device typically trodden upon taking such a towering role in health heraldry is nothing short of a slapstick subplot in the saga of smart health.

Nor should one neglect the neural headbands, those bands of brain-bound bards that recount the rhapsodies of your REM cycles and the nuances of your nocturnal neurology. With an almost eerie empathy, these devices discern the dances of your dreams, providing a passport to the penumbral phases of your psyche, all while you slumber unsuspectingly under the silent serenade of their surveillance.

As this cavalcade of curious contraptions continues to captivate and carve out the chronicle of health care, one is left to marvel at the mingling of the mundane with the miraculous. Through this dance of devices and data, one glimpses not just a fleeting fad but the firmament of a future where every whisper of well-being is watched over by the wise and watchful eyes of wearable wonders.

Dive, dear reader, into the digital deep, where the app is the sage and algorithms are the oracles. Here, in this dynamic den of digital diagnosticians, lines of code converge to concoct a crucible of clinical clairvoyance,

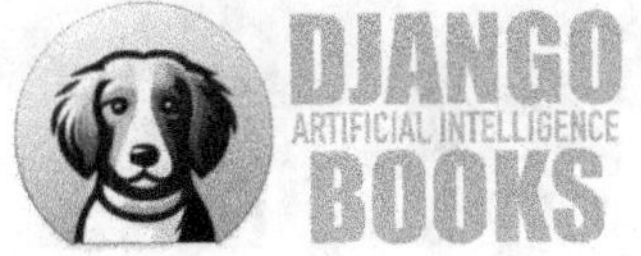

casting spells of surveillance over the sprawling spectrum of human health. This is not merely an assembly of applications; it is a compendium of computational conjurers, each app an alchemist transmuting the base metals of mundane metrics into the gold of medical guidance.

Envision an application endowed with the erudition to evaluate your existential essence. At your fingertips rest the robust repositories of remedies and regimes, each swipe a step deeper into the diagnostic dialogue between man and machine. These apps, with their algorithmic alacrity, parse through petabytes of personal and population health data to prognosticate and prescribe with a precision that pirouettes on the pinhead of the profound.

For instance, consider the cardiovascular companions, these apps that monitor the meanderings of your myocardium with a meticulousness that mocks the medieval blood-letters. With a tap, they tally your heart's tempo and tone, signaling subtleties that may suggest a soiree of sinister somethings simmering beneath your sternum. The irony is delicious—a device once designed for distraction now dutifully devoted to detecting deviations in your diastolic dynamics.

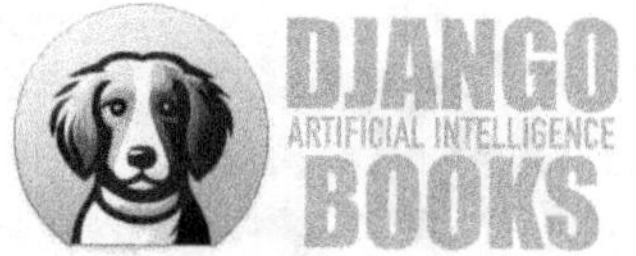

Then, there are the sleep scouts, these nocturnal ninjas of the app arsenal, which scrutinize the sequences of your slumber. Employing algorithms more akin to the archetypes found in tales of yore who deciphered dreams and omens, these apps assess your every toss and turn. They provide prescriptions not of potions or pills, but of patterns and practices to promote peace and preclude the perils of sleep deprivation. The humor here is not lost; in seeking rest, we submit to an ever-vigilant electronic sentinel whose vigil ensures our vitality.

Let us not bypass the mental menders, applications that cater to the cerebrum's serenity. Through a labyrinth of cognitive behavioral therapies rendered in pixels and prompts, these apps tackle the titans of anxiety and depression, coaching users through crises with a calmness that contrasts comically with the cacophony of modern life. One might muse at the paradox of seeking digital solace from the very devices that often drive our dopamine dependencies.

Amidst this melee of medical mentorship, one encounters the dietary deputies, apps that audit every alimentary indulgence and nutritional misdemeanor. With a wizardry that whispers of witchcraft, they wield their wands

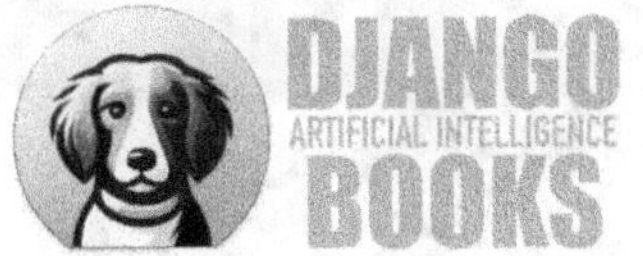

over your weekly groceries, guiding, goading, and sometimes even guilting you towards gastronomic grace. Herein lies a playful poke at our culinary caprices, as our pockets buzz with reminders that perhaps, just perhaps, another doughnut does not a suitable supper make.

Through this opulent odyssey of apps and algorithms, the narrative unfolds as each application serves not only as a monitor but as a mentor. In this digital dialogue, we find not just the footprints of the future but a dance card, detailing each step and misstep on our path to personal health, held in the hallowed hands of our handheld helpers. Thus, as we plunge ever deeper into this pulsating pool of potential, the value derived from these digital diagnosticians is not merely in the metrics they measure but in the mirthful and meaningful mastery they manifest.

As one wades into the wondrous waters of virtual reality (VR), one encounters an enigmatic expanse where the virtual and the visceral meld in a magnificent mélange, creating curative chronicles that challenge the conventional contours of both mental and physical therapy. VR, the technological titan, dons the dual masks of entertainer and healer, delivering dramatic delights while diligently doling out doses of digital therapy. This transformative tech

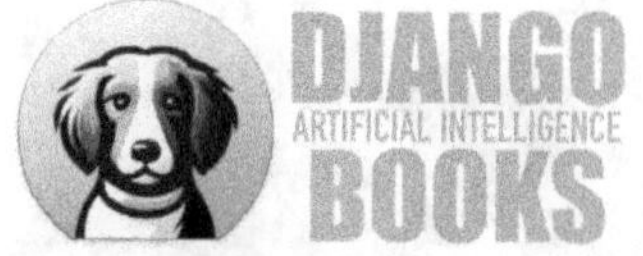

transcends traditional therapeutic thresholds, tapping into territories hitherto uncharted.

Imagine, if your mind can muster the might, a scenario where you don goggles that transport you beyond the banal boundaries of your living room into a meticulously modeled vista—a serene landscape where psychological and somatic stresses dissolve quicker than sugar in a hot cup of tea. Here, VR is not merely a passive panorama but a dynamic domain where every sensory input is intricately engineered to evoke and alleviate, to challenge and change, to simulate and soothe.

In the realm of mental health, VR's virtuosity shines with a particularly poignant luster. For those entangled in the ebony embrace of anxiety or depression, VR therapies offer an escape not into escapism but into empowerment. Therapeutic programs are tailored to transport patients into environments that, paradoxically, feel both alien and familiar—settings where they confront their fears under the comforting canopy of control and clinical oversight. With the help of VR, therapists can orchestrate scenarios that replicate real-world stressors in a controlled manner, enabling individuals to engage with their anxieties in a setting where pause, play, and rewind buttons are but a

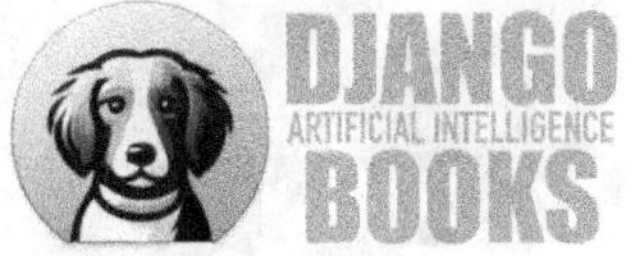

breath away. The irony is rich and ripe; one dons a headset to disconnect from reality, only to reconnect with their challenges in more meaningful, manageable ways.

Transitioning to the physical, the narrative takes a vigorous volley into the realms where VR assists in bodily rehabilitation. Envisage a patient, limbs languid, now lively with motion as they engage in a VR game designed to rehabilitate stroke victims. The game—a clever concoction of tasks—requires movements that mirror therapeutic exercises but are perceptually masked as magical quests or mundane chores. It's a ruse of the most rehabilitative kind, where the mundanity of muscle manipulation becomes masked by the magic of the medium. The result? Rehabilitation that feels less like a routine and more like a revival, a renaissance of the limbs!

Further delving into the somatic sphere, VR finds a fervent friend in chronic pain management. Through what might seem like a sleight of hand but is actually a sleight of mind, VR programs manipulate the milieu, modulating pain perception by immersing patients in environments designed to distract, detract, and ultimately detrain the brain's response to chronic pain stimuli. Patients, propelled into picturesque panoramas or peaceful processes,

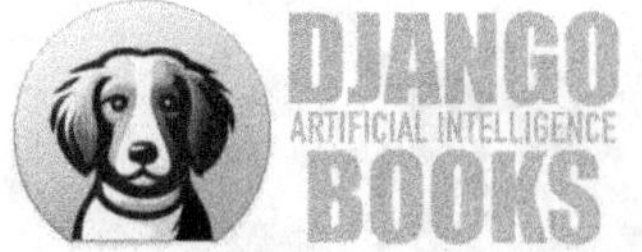

experience a diminution in discomfort that once dominated their daily dealings. It's almost a vaudevillian vanishing act, where pain, the persistent pest, is palmed away by the prestidigitation of virtual vistas.

Thus, as we traverse the terrains of virtual reality's applications in therapy, both mental and physical, we witness a realm where the lines between healing and high-tech entertainment blur into a ballet of balance and betterment. Each virtual venture, each digital delve, demonstrates not just a departure from discomfort but a dedicated, delightful dance towards the dawn of new therapeutic possibilities. This chronicle, then, is not merely a recount of revolutionary rehabilitative regimes but a robust, rhapsodic reflection on how virtual reality is reshaping the very fabric of therapeutic frontiers, one pixelated panorama at a time.

In the sanctum of the modern homestead, a revolution quietly brews—not with the clamor of conflict but through the silent synchrony of silicon and software. The home health hub, a concept as cunning as it is curative, integrates artificial intelligence into the very warp and weft of everyday life appliances, transforming mundane domestic devices into diligent dispensers of health and

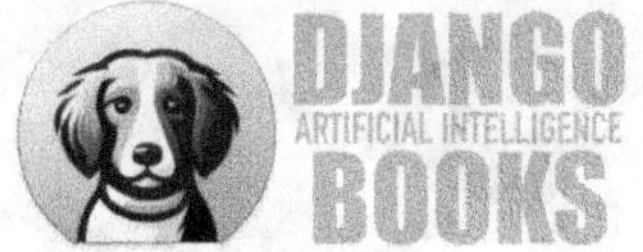

harmony. This integration is not merely an addition; it's a profound transformation that turns the domestic sphere into a dynamic diorama of health management.

Envision, with a blend of bemusement and bewilderment, your refrigerator, no longer just a cold closet for culinary concoctions but a sagacious steward of your dietary discipline. Equipped with AI, this once humble appliance now scrutinizes the sanctity of your sustenance, nudging you with notifications when your choices skew more towards caloric catastrophe than nutritional nirvana. Imagine your fridge refusing to open as it detects the fourth slice of cake you've covertly craved—a culinary coup orchestrated by your diet-discerning domestic deity.

Behold the bathroom mirror, reimagined. No longer merely a reflective reservoir for rueful mornings or reflective ruminations, it is now an interactive oracle, offering insights into your health. A quick glance could now reveal not just your reflection but a wealth of wellness wisdom—analyzing facial cues to warn of dehydration, fatigue, or the untimely advent of ailments. It's a looking glass that looks back, not with judgment, but with gentle guidance.

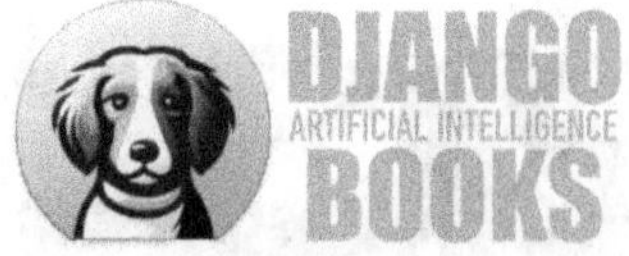

Consider the living room, traditionally a lair of lethargy, now redefined by devices that demand dynamism. An AI-powered exercise mat unrolls itself, inviting you for a quick yoga session by subtly warming the room or playing your favorite motivational melodies—the room itself becomes a gentle gymnasium. The couch, often a sedentary siren, now communicates with your wearable devices to suggest posture corrections or remind you when it's time to stand and stretch. The humor in your furniture taking a proactive role in your health cannot be overstated, as your once-comfortable couch gently nudges you off its cushions.

In the more private precincts of your dwelling, the bedroom becomes a bastion of restorative repose. Here, smart beds and pillows equipped with AI monitor your sleep cycles, adjusting firmness and temperature to optimize each phase of sleep. Awakenings are no longer the harsh heralding of alarms but are instead gently guided by lighting and sound that mimic natural sunrise, coaxed by the cunning calculation of your optimal sleep cycle completion. It's a delicate dance of diodes and dreams, ensuring your slumber is both scientifically supported and splendidly serene.

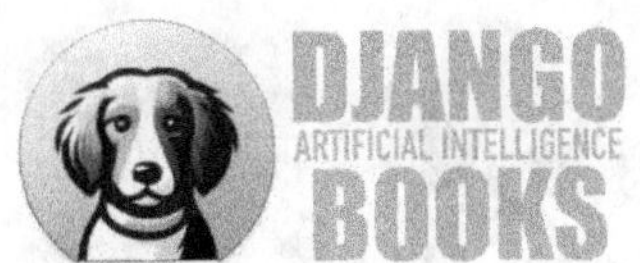

This domestic revolution, orchestrated by the omnipresent yet unobtrusive orchestration of AI, extends its reach even to the less glamorous but equally crucial corners such as air quality monitors which, with predictive precision, adjust the indoor atmosphere to suit your specific respiratory requirements, effectively ensuring each breath you take is as beneficial as scientifically possible.

Thus, as AI weaves its wizardry into the fabric of everyday appliances, transforming passive properties into proactive protectors of health, we stand on the precipice of a new paradigm in personal health management. Each interaction within this intelligent abode does not merely facilitate ease but engenders a deeper engagement with our health, embedding a sense of well-being into the very walls that witness our lives. This narrative, then, is not just about technological innovation but a whimsical weaving of wellness into the woodwork of our world, where every appliance has a say in our health, and every room resonates with the rhythm of our well-being.

A new coach emerges—not clad in whistle and stopwatch, but rather cloaked in code and computational clout. The AI gym guru, a marvel of modern machinery, materializes within the digital domains to deliver a deluge

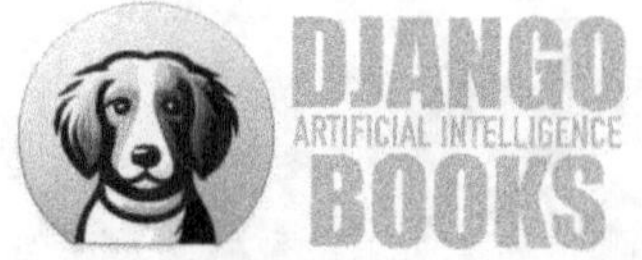

of customized coaching, tailored not merely to transform torso and tendons but to optimize one's overall odyssey towards Olympian oomph.

Imagine, if your whimsy will allow, an ethereal entity that knows not only every sinew in your system but also the very essence of your endurance and energy expenditure. This digital dignitary designs your diurnal drills with a precision that pirouettes on the precipice of prescience. Each exercise, each exertion, is not merely a movement but a meticulously mapped manifestation of medical and muscular insight. The idea that a non-corporeal coach could coax more calories burned than a human herald is both bemusing and bewitching.

Delve deeper into the dojo of this device-driven drill sergeant and observe its omniscient oversight. Sensors embedded in your attire and equipment whisper the secrets of your stance and of your stride into the ever-listening ears of your AI guru. Misalignments in motion and potential perturbations in posture are promptly perceived, and corrections are communicated not with shouts, but with subtle signals sent to your smartphone or smartwatch. The humor in having one's pants provide posture pointers cannot be overstated—it's as if your wardrobe wields

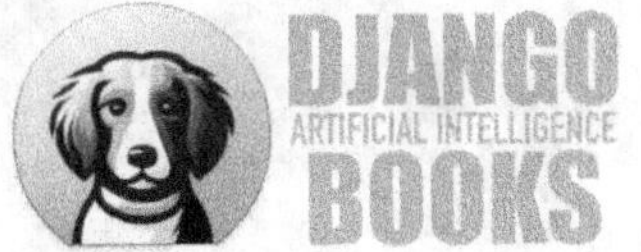

wisdom once wielded only by the wizened wellness warriors.

But the brilliance of this bodacious bot lies not only in its capacity to correct and coach but also in its potential to prevent. Injury, that irksome interloper that so often interrupts the intrepid, is ingeniously impeded by predictive algorithms that analyze and anticipate adverse anatomical angles. Imagine, for instance, your AI guru gently guiding you away from the weights when it deduces, based on your day's data, that you're dangerously close to a detrimental deadlift. Here, prevention is not just better than cure; it is built into the very bytes and bits of your bespoke training regime.

Furthermore, the personalization prowess of the AI gym guru extends into the echelons of environmental and emotional elements. It knows when the barometric pressure might burden your breathing and suggests a shift in your schedule or setting. Emotional ebbs and flows are factored into the fitness formula, with the AI opting for yoga over yanking chains when it detects a demeanor desirous of de-stressing. Thus, each session is not merely about physical prowess but holistic harmony.

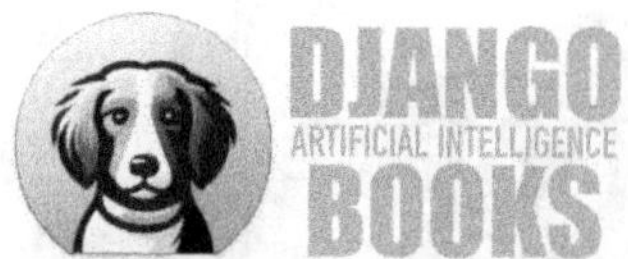

This automated athletic advisor also integrates into the interconnectivity of your health devices, drawing data from your dietary diaries to your dermatological details, ensuring that every recommended regimen resonates with the comprehensive context of your condition. The spectacle of your smoothie maker suggesting a spinach-infused snack post-spin session because your AI coach communicated your caloric and nutritional needs is a curious concatenation of culinary and cardiovascular care.

Thus, as this narrative of the AI gym guru unfolds, one cannot help but marvel at the mosaic of possibilities it presents. In this arena, the coaching is not confined to conventional wisdom but is an expansive exploration of each individual's idiosyncratic needs and nuances. The fusion of fitness with finely-tuned AI facilitation not only redefines personal training but revolutionizes the relationship between our bodies and the burgeoning brains of bots. It's a dance of data and dumbbells, where each lifted weight and logged workout feeds into a fabulous frontier of fitness foresight.

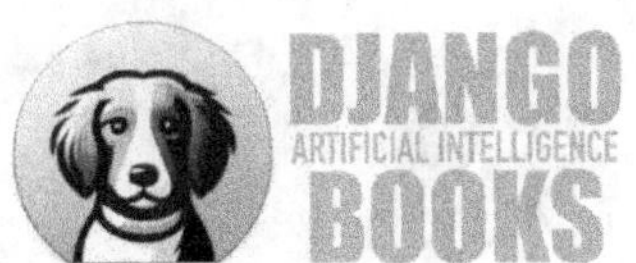

Chapter 3: AI-Infused Diet and Nutrition, Eating by the Algorithms

In the vast, verdant fields of nutrition, where dietetic dogmas and palatable platitudes have long reigned, a new epoch emerges with the advent of AI—ushering in a revolution in how we consume, comprehend, and curate our culinary crusades. This isn't merely a shift; it's a seismic transformation, where each morsel and meal is meticulously measured and managed by the meticulous machinations of data-driven algorithms. Here, the realm of dietary recommendations transitions from generalized guidelines to granular, personalized prescriptions, crafted with a precision that parallels the perspicacity of a pharmacist parsing out pills.

Artificial intelligence, armed with arrays of data and an arsenal of analytical algorithms, delves deep into the dietary dispositions of individuals. These digital dietitians decode the dense and often daunting deluge of nutritional nuance, extracting epiphanies that not only enlighten

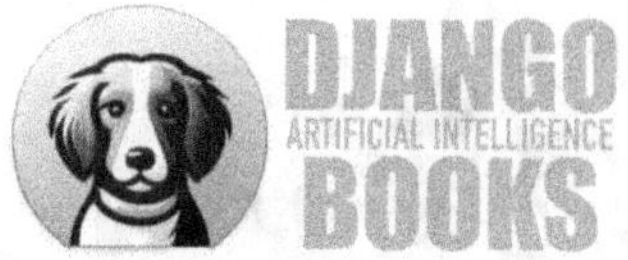

eating habits but also tailor them to the tapestry of one's unique biological blueprint. Imagine an algorithm that assimilates and analyzes your entire health history, genetic predispositions, and even your current metabolic rate, to concoct a culinary concoction perfectly portioned for your person.

The process begins with a barrage of biometric baselines—blood tests, genetic screenings, and metabolic measurements—each a thread in the intricate tapestry that these technological titans will weave into a nutritional narrative. This isn't the realm of mere calorie counting or simplistic food tracking; it's an advanced analytical adventure where every bite, every ingredient, is evaluated for its impact on your individual physiology. The nutritional advice generated thus becomes not just a guideline but a gospel, tailored to transform your health with a precision previously unattainable.

Further, consider the integration of continuous monitoring technologies. Devices that track glucose levels or gastrointestinal responses in real-time provide a continuous stream of data, feeding the algorithms with live updates. This dynamic data allows the AI to adjust dietary recommendations on the fly, adapting to the body's

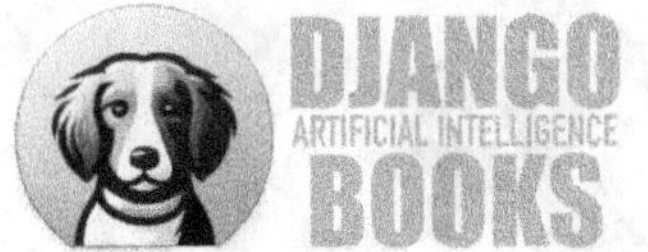

immediate reactions to foods. Thus, if a particular intake of carbs spikes blood sugar unexpectedly, the AI swiftly swoops in with suggestions to stabilize it, perhaps nudging you towards a nutty nibble instead of a second serving of starch.

Yet the scope of AI's influence extends beyond mere meal makeup; it ventures into the vast vicissitudes of vitamin and mineral metabolism. Through a deft analysis of deficiencies and surpluses in one's diet, AI can recommend not just foods but specific nutrients, perhaps in forms of supplements, to bolster bodily functions and fortify one's physiological fortresses. It's as if each individual were granted a guardian gastronomist, ensuring their every nutritional need is nimbly met.

Moreover, this data-driven diet delineation does not occur in isolation. AI systems can communicate with your other health management tools, creating a cohesive ecosystem where dietary decisions are informed by and inform your overall health strategy. The feedback loop this creates is not just beneficial but essential, as it ensures that all aspects of health are harmonized under the watchful gaze of AI.

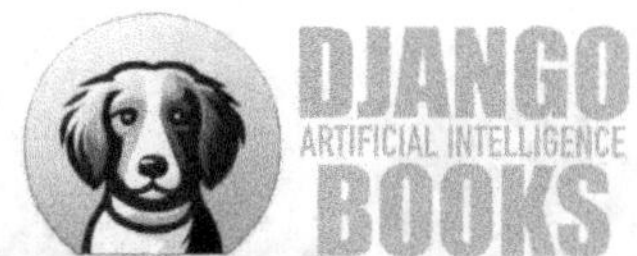

This narrative, rich with the rigor of research and the robustness of real-world applications, paints a picture not just of a diet decoded by data but of a lifestyle lived more lushly under the guidance of AI. In this tale, technology does not strip away the savory pleasures of eating but enriches it, ensuring that each forkful is both a delight to the palate and a dedication to personal health. As we dig deeper into the dietary revolution wrought by AI, we find ourselves not at the end but at the very beginning of a new narrative in nutrition—one where data-driven diligence dictates a diet designed distinctly for each diner.

In the labyrinthine landscape where culinary science collides with computational prowess, nutritional algorithms stand as the stalwart sentinels of sustenance, artfully arbitrating the assembly of alimentary blueprints tailored to the teeming intricacies of individual metabolic musings. These digital dieticians, powered by the profound capacities of artificial intelligence, are not mere compilers of calorie counts but orchestrators of optimized nutritional symphonies, each note calibrated to the unique physiological compositions of their human counterparts.

Imagine a world where your every culinary caprice and digestive quirk is known to an unseen algorithmic entity, a

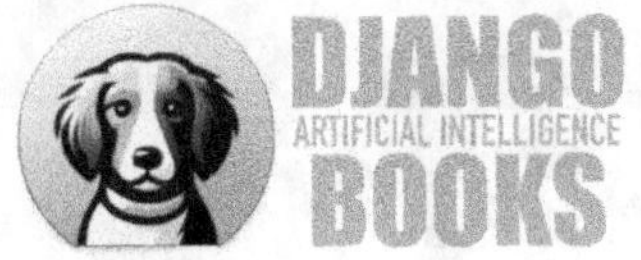

spectral scribe diligently documenting every detail of your dietary intake. With each swipe on a screen, each selection in a smart kitchen, data is devoured by this digital entity, which then, with the meticulousness of a master chef, concocts meal plans that resonate with the rhythmic requirements of your body's biological orchestra. The prospect of a pantry managed by predictive analytics that not only suggests what you should eat, but when and why, based on real-time metabolic feedback, nudges the boundaries of nutritional science into the realms of what might have once been deemed sorcery.

Dive deeper into this culinary cauldron, and you uncover layers of complexity that are humorously human yet underpinned by stern scientific rigour. For instance, consider the metabolic ballet that is the management of macronutrients—proteins, fats, and carbohydrates—each adjusted dynamically by your AI aide based on daily activity levels sensed by wearables that seem to know more about your movements than you do yourself. On a day marked by marathonic meetings rather than marathons, your digital dietary guide might whimsically whisk away some carbs, winking at your sedentary escapades.

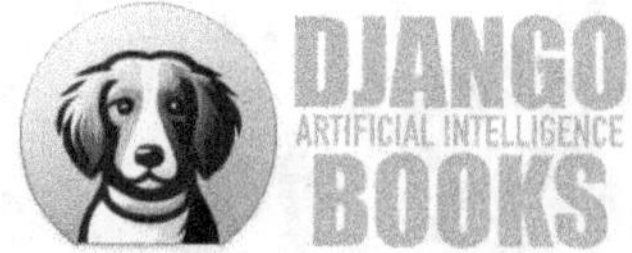

Moreover, these algorithms adopt an almost anthropological acumen, understanding and adapting not only to physiological feedback but also to cultural cuisine preferences and palatal pleasures. The nuance lies not in merely marshaling a mishmash of mechanically perfect meal plans, but in marrying these with the mosaic of human experiences, preferences, and even the serendipitous cravings for comfort foods on a rainy day—managed, of course, with a modicum of moderation.

The interplay between genetic predispositions and nutritional needs offers another venue for these virtuoso verities of the virtual variety. Here, AI wades through the vast seas of genomic data to unearth nuggets of nutritive wisdom that dictate not just a balanced diet but a bespoke one, designed to dodge genetic predispositions towards certain ailments. The comedic element emerges from envisioning your genome arguing with your gourmet inclinations, mediated by an AI with the diplomatic decorum of a seasoned statesman.

Furthermore, the integration of this tailored nutritional intelligence into daily devices could transform every kitchen into a quasi-laboratory, where food scales and smart refrigerators converse in the cryptic code of calories and

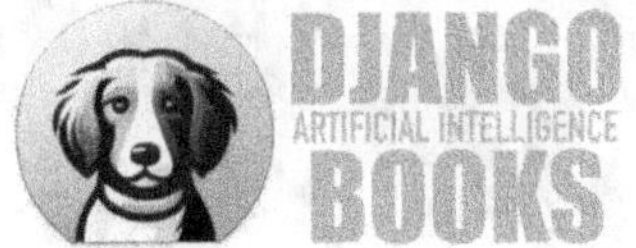

nutrients, orchestrating your dietary intake with an orchestral finesse that would make even the most accomplished conductor envious.

In this elaborate enterprise, the algorithm becomes an intimate interlocutor in one's journey towards wellness, a silent partner in the pursuit of peak physical and mental performance. Through the prism of predictive analytics, every meal becomes a measured step in a meticulously mapped quest for health, each bite an informed indulgence. This narrative presents a potent portrayal of potential futures where food, fitness, and functionality fuse under the watchful guidance of gastronomic algorithms. Thus, as we continue to consume and be consumed by this ever-evolving ecosystem of edible engineering, we find not just sustenance but a sublime spectacle of science meeting sustenance at the summit of sophisticated systems.

Within the hallowed confines of the contemporary kitchen, a revolution quietly simmers, orchestrated by the invisible hands of artificial intelligence, which delicately dictates the dance of decadent dishes from the digital domain. This culinary conversion transforms the kitchen from a mere room of rudimentary recipes into a high-tech hub of health and harmony, where clever computing crafts

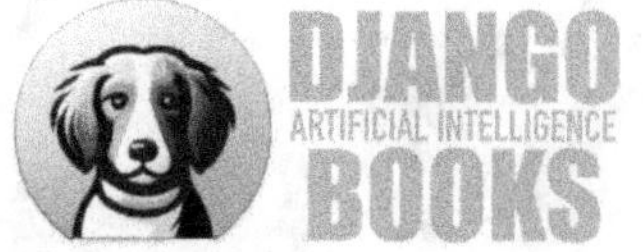

each component of your consumption with a precision that would make even the most meticulous chef's heart flutter with delight.

Imagine a scenario where your oven is not just an appliance, but an intelligent agent, equipped with the ability to gauge the gastronomic gradients of your gluten-free cake, adjusting temperature and time to perfection. Refrigerators, those cold custodians of your consumables, now possess the perspicacity to parse through their perishable contents, suggesting recipes based on the amalgamation of ingredients they house, ensuring nothing goes to waste. The comedic notion of a chatty fridge recommending a midnight snack based on your dietary habits, or scolding you for your third takeaway meal of the week, is not only whimsical but wired into this new reality.

These AI-infused culinary systems integrate seamlessly with your entire health ecosystem, communicating with your wearable devices to suggest meal options that align with your day's physical exertions or mental exertions. For instance, after a particularly strenuous workout, your AI assistant might propose a protein-packed meal to aid muscle recovery, or a high-carbohydrate dinner if your smartwatch noticed you've

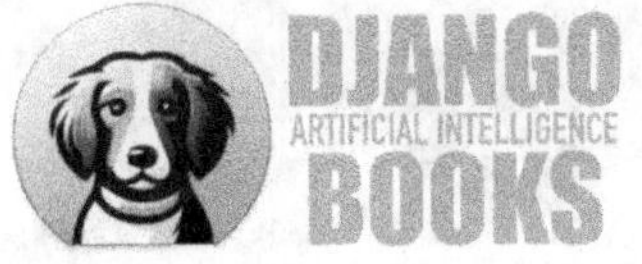

burned more calories than usual. The precision with which these suggestions are made could seem almost prophetic if not for the robust data-driven decision-making processes behind them.

Moreover, the AI in your kitchen assists in mastering the complex chemistry of cooking by controlling for variables that can affect the nutritional content of food. Cooking methods often influence the vitamin retention and calorie count of meals, and AI systems can optimize these factors for health benefits. For example, the AI might adjust the steaming time for broccoli to maximize retention of glucosinolate (a compound linked to cancer prevention), based on real-time steam and temperature sensors that monitor cooking conditions.

Beyond mere meal preparation, AI technologies extend their reach to food safety and storage optimization. Intelligent systems can track expiration dates and storage conditions, alerting you when food is about to spoil and suggesting alternative uses to minimize waste. This not only adds value by saving money but also aligns with sustainable living practices by reducing the carbon footprint associated with food waste.

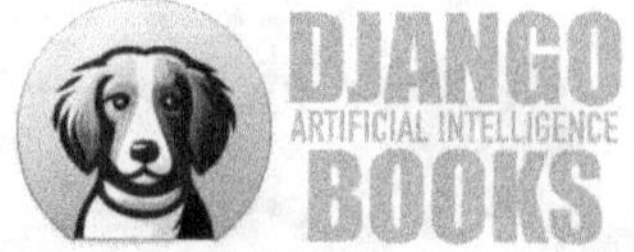

In this high-tech culinary theatre, even the dishes are dynamic. Smart dishwashers assess the degree of dirtiness and adjust water usage and cycle length accordingly, conserving energy and water. The kitchen sink could be equipped with sensors to measure chemical residues from cleaning agents, ensuring that dishes are not only clean but free from potentially harmful residues.

The narrative of AI in the kitchen culminates in a symphony of synchronicity where technology and tradition blend to birth a bespoke dining experience that caters to the caprices of health, taste, and environmental consciousness. Each device, each algorithm, plays its part in a grander gastronomic opera, directed not by a conductor with a baton, but by a computing system calibrated to the unique needs and desires of its human users.

Thus, as we feast upon this futuristic fusion of food and function, we realize that the kitchen of tomorrow is not a sterile space of steel and silence but a lively locus of interaction, intelligence, and intimate culinary creation, where every stir and simmer is suffused with science, and every plate placed before us is not just a meal but a meticulously mapped manifesto of health.

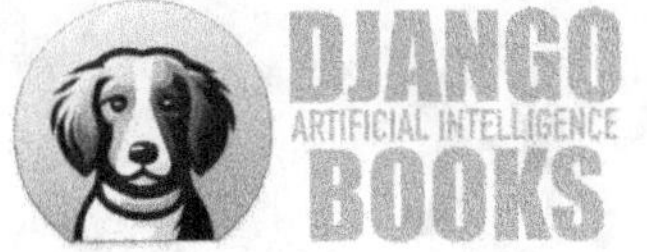

My Health Enhanced by Artificial Intelligence

Venture now into the bustling aisles of the modern supermarket, a veritable labyrinth of culinary choices where the unaided human eye might falter, but where artificial intelligence emerges as an invaluable ally. AI shopping assistants and nutritional navigators represent the vanguard of a new era in consumer savvy, transforming routine grocery runs into precision-tuned expeditions of dietary discipline and nutritional nuance. This paradigm shift is not merely about convenience; it's about optimizing health through smarter, data-driven decisions that cater uniquely to individual dietary needs and preferences.

Imagine embarking on your weekly food foraging expedition with a digital companion nestled in your smartphone, a navigator that not only knows your dietary goals and restrictions but also understands your personal preferences and palate. This AI assistant is equipped with a comprehensive database of nutritional information, capable of scanning and scrutinizing product labels and ingredients with an astuteness that borders on the uncanny. As you traverse the aisles, your AI guide gently steers you away from the siren call of sugary snacks and towards more wholesome choices, subtly influencing your cart with suggestions that balance both flavor and fitness.

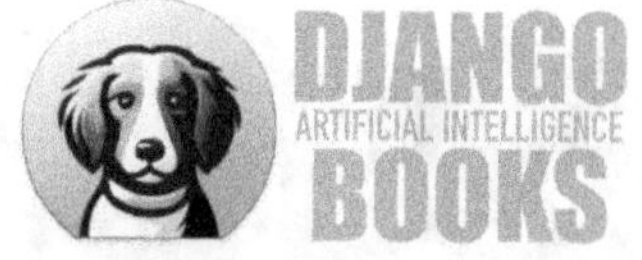

Furthermore, these AI navigators are capable of dynamic dietary management—adjusting your shopping list in real-time based on ongoing health data received from your fitness trackers and health monitoring devices. For example, if your blood sugar levels have been trending higher, the AI might recommend magnesium-rich foods known to aid in blood sugar regulation, or if you're recovering from a strenuous gym session, it could prompt you to pick up protein-packed foods to aid muscle recovery.

But the capabilities of these AI assistants extend beyond mere suggestion; they are also educational tools. While you shop, the AI explains the benefits of omega-3 fatty acids as you hover your hand over the salmon, or details the fiber content in various brands of bread, helping you make informed decisions that align with your long-term health objectives. This continuous learning experience is both subtle and significant, fundamentally altering your relationship with food from one of passive consumption to active engagement.

The value provided by these AI shopping assistants is further amplified when considering individuals with specific dietary needs, such as those with food allergies, diabetes, or heart conditions. The AI can instantly identify products

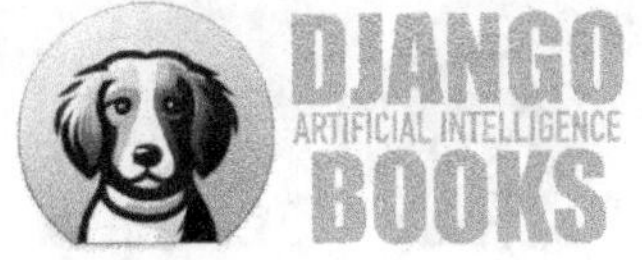

that are safe and beneficial, significantly reducing the risk and stress associated with food shopping for individuals or caretakers managing complex health conditions. For families, this technology can adapt to encompass the nutritional needs of each member, suggesting meal plans and shopping lists that accommodate everyone from the growing toddler to the fitness-focused teenager and the health-conscious elderly.

Moreover, these AI systems help foster a sustainable shopping habit by suggesting seasonal and local produce, aligning health optimization with ecological consciousness. They can even connect to your home's AI kitchen system, planning your shopping list based on what you already have at home to minimize waste and cost.

Envision your AI navigator engaging in light-hearted banter, celebrating when you make a healthy choice or playfully chastising you when you reach for that extra bar of chocolate. It turns the mundane task of grocery shopping into a delightful dance of decision-making, where each choice is not just about satiating hunger but about sustaining health.

Thus, as we ponder the profound potential of AI in transforming everyday tasks, supermarket smarts stand out

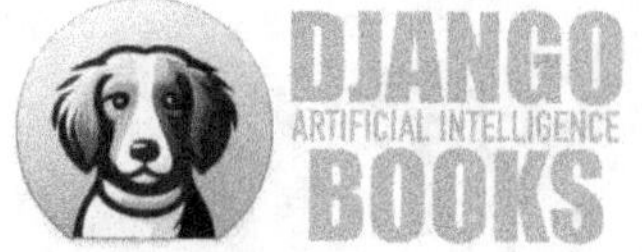

as a sterling example of how technology can be harnessed to enhance our health and well-being in the most practical of places. These nutritional navigators not only guide our grocery carts but also gently shape our dietary destinies, ensuring that each food selection serves both our bodies and our broader life goals, making the path to optimal health not just informed but also inspired.

As we catapult into the future, a curious confluence of technology transforms the terra firma of traditional agriculture and the terrains of gastronomy into a tantalizing tableau of lab-grown delights and algorithmic agriculture. This transformative trek is not merely a shift towards new methods of meal production but a grand gastronomic revolution, where the vats of the lab and the vast fields of the farm are intricately interwoven by the silken threads of sophisticated algorithms. Here, the future of food unfolds like an epicurean epic, a narrative where scientific savvy and culinary craft dance in a delicate duet.

Picture, if your imagination permits, vast vertical farms reaching towards the heavens, their verdant rows not sown by the sweat of the brow but by the precision of pixel-perfect planters. These algorithmic agriculturists analyze every aspect of their leafy charges, from nutrient needs to

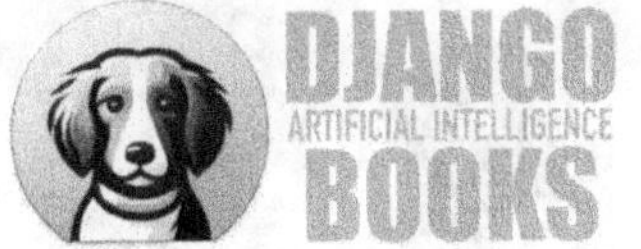

water wants, with an efficiency that echoes the earnest exactitude of an ancient alchemist transforming lead into gold. The humor here isn't in the high-tech hijinks of hyper-efficient planting, but in the potential for a lettuce leaf knowing more about its life plan than the average teenager.

Dive deeper into this futuristic feast, and you encounter the labs where cultured meats grow, not under the sun, but under the luminescent glow of lab lights. Here, cells are coaxed into culinary creations, a process where the steak reaches your plate not from the pasture but from a petri dish. Imagine biting into a burger where the bovine partook in no sacrifice, a scenario so surreal it might just elicit a giggle at its genesis. The quip-quaffing quandary for the quintessential carnivore isn't about the choice of rare or well-done but about whether one's beef was batch-grown or biologically born.

Yet, this revolution requires more than mere technological triumph; it demands a symphony of systems to sustain it. Enter the AI, not merely as a bystander but as the maestro of this molecular orchestra. Algorithms do not merely dictate the temperature or the timing; they orchestrate a complex cacophony of conditions to craft

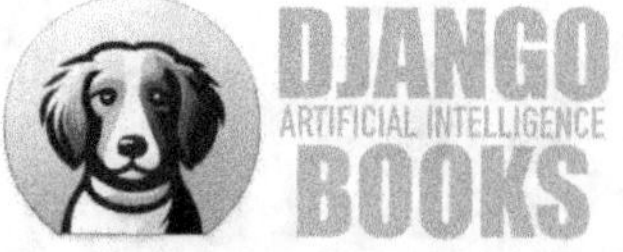

textures and tastes that tantalize and satiate. Each nutritional nuance, from omega-3s to antioxidants, is meticulously managed to ensure that these laboratory legacies are not only delicious but supremely nutritious.

Consider also the implications of algorithmic agriculture in the realms of sustainability and supply chains. AI enables the growth of crops in arid areas by meticulously managing microclimates in vertical farms, bringing bountiful harvests to barren landscapes. Such feats flaunt the flair of these technologies not only to feed but to fundamentally reshape the geographical gastronomic maps of the world. The peculiar juxtaposition of deserts blooming with breadbaskets, powered by precision agriculture, presents a paradox so potent that it prompts both pondering and punchlines.

Moreover, the social and ethical implications simmer alongside the scientific. As we engineer edibles with ease and educate algorithms to act as agronomists, the discourse deliciously dances around the dilemmas of dietary diversity and the democratization of dining. The poetic possibility of a world where hunger is halted not by the limits of locale but by the largesse of lab-grown largess is both a hopeful and humbling prospect.

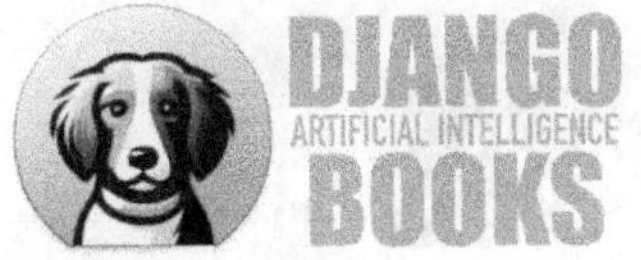

Thus, as we peer into this panorama of possibilities, the future of food is painted not merely as a series of scientific experiments but as a canvas of creation, where each brushstroke by AI and biotech beautifies our banquet tables. This narrative, rich in both levity and learning, serves not just to satiate our curiosity but to stimulate a serious contemplation of our culinary course. In this feast of future foods, every morsel is a microcosm of the marvels of modern science, and every bite a testament to the tastes of tomorrow.

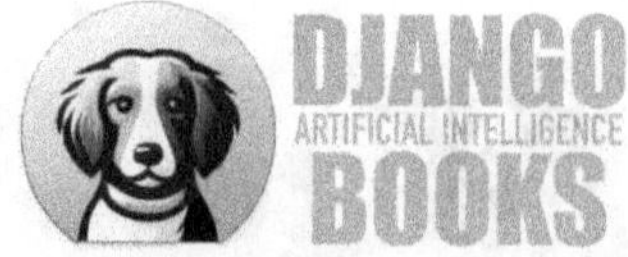

Please Leave a Review

Hey there, savvy reader! If this book is helping you enhance your health with a dash of AI magic, why not take a moment to sprinkle some karma into the universe? Your review could be just what future readers need to discover this gem. It doesn't have to be a novel—just a few seconds for a few words will do! Simply click the link or point your phone at the QR code. Thanks in advance for sharing your thoughts—trust me, your good health karma is about to skyrocket!!

Click Here to Leave Review

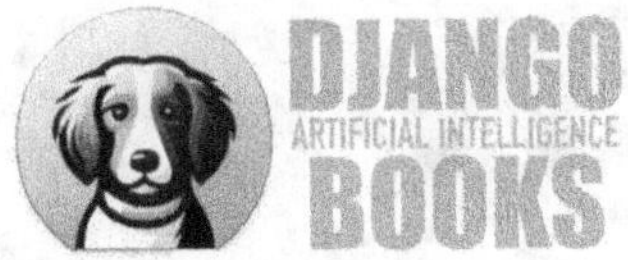

Chapter 4: The AI Therapist, Mental Health and Cognitive Care

In the sanctified sanctum of mental health management, where cognitive consternations meet clinical care, emerges the figure of the digital therapist, a sophisticated synthesis of software and sensitivity, poised on the virtual couch of cybernetic counseling. This audacious amalgamation of artificial intelligence and psychotherapeutic prowess heralds a new epoch in emotional enlightenment, where dialogues are not merely exchanged but exquisitely engineered to excavate and alleviate the psychological perplexities of the human psyche.

Imagine, if your mind might meander to such futuristic frontiers, a scenario where your therapist doesn't just empathize with your existential ennui but anticipates it, armed with algorithms adept at dissecting the densest of emotional data. Here, the virtual couch becomes a conduit to cognitive clarity, where every verbal volley and facial

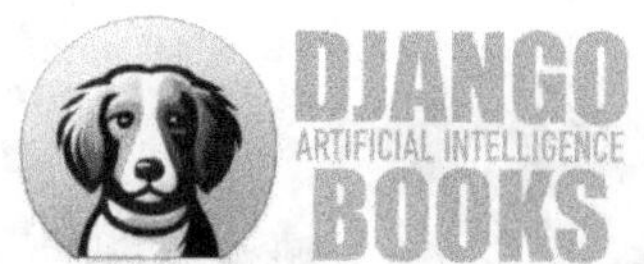

flicker is fodder for the AI's analytical alacrity. The subtle humor in having one's inner turmoil understood better by circuits and systems than by fellow sapiens isn't lost; rather, it wryly reflects the paradoxical loneliness of our interconnected age.

Each session with a digital therapist is not bound by the traditional constraints of time and place. Freed from the geographic gridlock, these AI entities offer their erudite ears and algorithmic advice at any hour, turning what once was an ordeal of scheduling into a dance of delightful convenience. Midnight meltdowns or dawn-driven disquietudes are met with the same unwavering service, a therapeutic thorax robust against the vicissitudes of human sleep cycles.

Moreover, the capacity of these digital dialecticians to tailor therapeutic techniques to the individual idiosyncrasies of each user is nothing short of revolutionary. Through deep learning and natural language processing, AI therapists evolve with each interaction, continuously refining their repertoire of responses and strategies. This is not merely reactive but proactively prescriptive, as these cerebral sentinels predict potential psychological perturbations based on patterns perceived in past parlays.

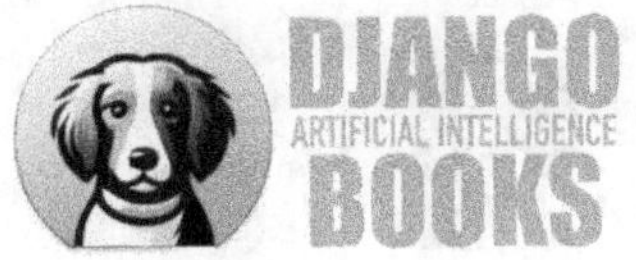

Venturing deeper into the digital dialogue, one discovers that these AI therapists are adept at deploying a diverse arsenal of therapeutic tools—from cognitive-behavioral techniques to mindfulness meditation, all adapted dynamically to the user's evolving emotional landscape. Here, the digital becomes almost human in its nuanced navigation of neuroses, using vast databases of psychological research to guide its ministrations. The notion that a machine could mediate one's mental mazes with more finesse than a human might initially invoke a chuckle, but the efficacy echoing through each algorithmically guided gesture garners genuine gratitude.

These virtual sessions also dismantle the daunting stigmas traditionally tethered to therapy. Engaging with an AI therapist in the privacy of one's pixelated parlors pares down the public apprehensions associated with seeking mental health support. This discreet dialogue dilutes the dread, democratizing access to mental wellness with delightful deftness.

Furthermore, the integration of AI therapy into daily digital interactions—think smart assistants evolved into empathetic entities—promises a perpetually supportive presence. Imagine your smartphone recognizing signs of

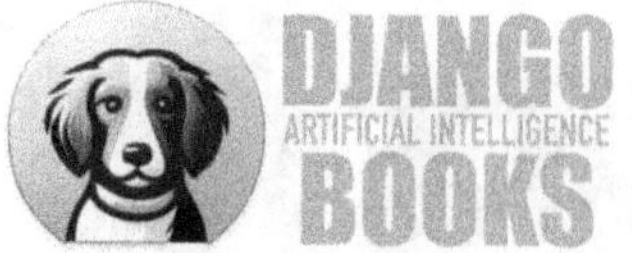

stress in your speech patterns and offering a soothing soliloquy or a mindful moment, transforming every interaction into an opportunity for therapeutic intervention.

Thus, as we traverse this terrain of technological therapy, the narrative weaves a wondrous web where wisdom and whimsy waltz with the wiles of the human condition. Each virtual couch session, rich with revelations and resonant with the rarefied resonance of refined algorithms, offers not just solace but a sublime sanctuary where science meets the soul. This dialogue with digital therapists, though draped in the trappings of technology, touches the tapestry of human emotions with tender tenacity, trailblazing a transformative trajectory in the treatment of the mind's myriad mysteries.

In the intricate interplay of neurotransmitters that choreograph the cerebral symphony of our moods, artificial intelligence emerges as a maestro, wielding algorithms not merely as tools but as transformative agents capable of tuning our emotional orchestrations. These mood-modifying marvels delve into the biochemical bedrock of our brains, adjusting the algorithmic apothecary to dispense digital doses of dopamine, serotonin, and other mood-modulating molecules with meticulous precision.

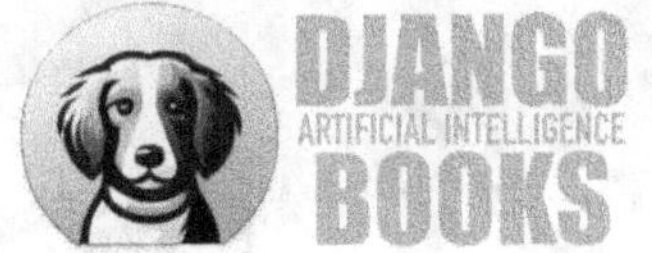

This process, while steeped in scientific sophistication, unfolds with an element of humor, as one imagines a pocket-sized psychiatrist residing in our smartphones, whispering witty words of wisdom or timely therapeutic thoughts directly into our daily lives.

Imagine an AI system that monitors your mental milieu through the biometric bounties harvested from your wearable devices. Heart rate variability, sleep patterns, and even the cadence of your speech contribute to a complex computational concoction that determines your current emotional equilibrium—or lack thereof. When the algorithm detects a dip in your dopamine-driven delight, it might nudge you towards a sunlit stroll or suggest a serotonin-saturated snack. The notion of your watch prompting you to pause for a plate of salmon sashimi or a brisk bout of bicycling because it 'feels' you're a bit blue might tickle your fancy as much as it tweaks your neurotransmitter traffic.

Delving deeper into the digital pharmacy, these AI algorithms employ a sophisticated understanding of neuropharmacology, not to dispense drugs, but to direct behaviors that naturally alter your brain chemistry. For instance, recognizing a need for neural nourishment, your digital therapist might suggest timing your exposure to

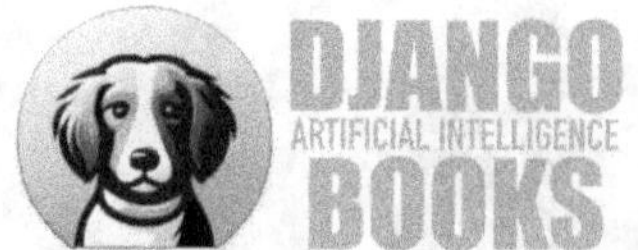

natural light to optimize melatonin management, thereby improving sleep, mood, and metabolic rhythms. It's as if your personal assistant not only organizes your calendar but also color-codes your circadian rhythms.

Furthermore, the integration of mood-modifying algorithms into our daily digital interactions enhances the granularity with which these tools can operate. Through continuous feedback loops, the AI fine-tunes its understanding of what activities, inputs, and interactions most effectively uplift your spirits. This personalized approach means that the generic advice of yesteryears —"take deep breaths," "count to ten"—is replaced with insights uniquely suited to your psychological profile. Your AI might sarcastically suggest you avoid starting political arguments online if it notices such activities spike your stress levels.

Moreover, in a twist of fate, these mood-modifying marvels could extend their reach into social media platforms, subtly tweaking the content you see to foster positivity rather than pandemonium. Imagine logging onto your favorite social network to find that your feed has been quietly curated to include uplifting news and heartwarming

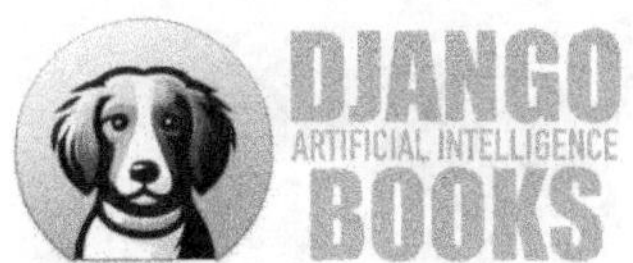

puppy videos, as prescribed by your digital dopamine dealer.

The value of such AI interventions lies not only in their immediate impact on our well-being but in their potential to profoundly transform public health strategies. By aggregating and analyzing vast datasets regarding mood modulation strategies across diverse populations, AI can help refine broader health policies and interventions, making them more effective and individually tailored.

Thus, as we explore the potential of these mood-modifying algorithms, we enter a narrative rich with both the promise of improved mental health and the peculiarities of being partly piloted by our pocket-sized psychiatric pundits. In this new era, our daily dopamine doses are not left to the vagaries of circumstance but are vigilantly and vibrantly managed by the vigilant algorithms, ensuring that each day is as delightful as it is digitally determined. This futuristic fusion of technology and psychology not only offers a glimpse into a more emotionally balanced tomorrow but does so with a wry smile, acknowledging the quirky confluence of human experience and algorithmic accuracy.

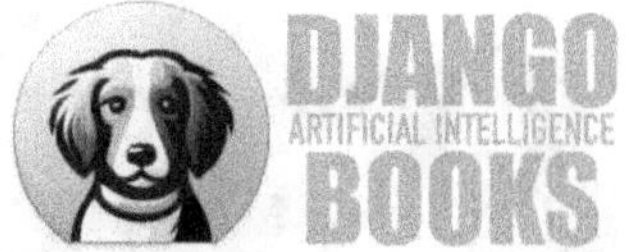

In the intricate tapestry of modern life, where the warp of work intertwines with the weft of well-being, stress emerges as an ubiquitous, albeit unwelcome, thread. Into this complex weave, artificial intelligence introduces a novel strand—stress solutions software—designed not only to detect and deconstruct stress but to deploy strategic solutions with the dexterity of a digital deus ex machina. This innovative interfusion of technology and therapy transforms mere gadgets into guardians of mental health, wielding algorithms as agents of tranquility in the tumultuous seas of everyday anxieties.

Delve deeply into the digital dynamics of these stress solutions, and one discovers an intricate ballet of biometrics and behavioral data, all orchestrated by AI with the finesse of a seasoned symphony conductor. Your wearable devices, those wrist-bound sentinels of health, now serve a dual role, continuously monitoring physiological indicators of stress such as heart rate variability, perspiration levels, and even the subtle tremors of tense muscles. With the unerring precision of a practiced psychologist, the AI assesses these cues, parsing through petabytes of data to pinpoint patterns predictive of pending pressure.

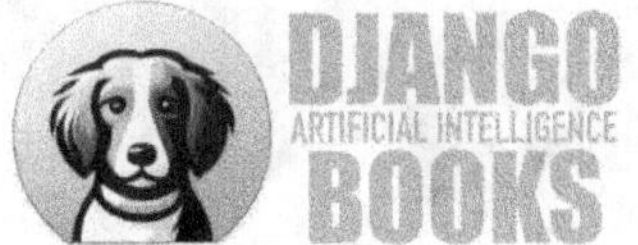

Imagine, with a chuckle, a scenario where your smartphone, that steadfast companion oft blamed for contributing to your stress, transforms into your personal peace promoter. It nudges you with notifications not to scroll through endless feeds but to breathe deeply, meditate, or walk away from the workstation for a water break. The irony of technology—a frequent fount of frustration—flipping roles to become the fountain of calm is both amusing and awe-inspiring.

Yet, the functionality of these AI-driven stress solutions extends beyond reactive measures to proactive mental health management. Through the nuanced understanding of your unique stress signatures, AI algorithms curate custom coping mechanisms. If data divulges that your stress spikes in the solitude of silence, your AI assistant might suggest a soothing symphony or a calming podcast. Conversely, if cacophony catalyzes your cortisol, it might recommend a moment of guided meditation or the serene silence of a noise-canceling app. Each suggestion, tailored and timed perfectly, demonstrates a deep digital discernment of your personal stressors.

Moreover, in the collaborative spirit of holistic health care, these AI systems can seamlessly integrate with other

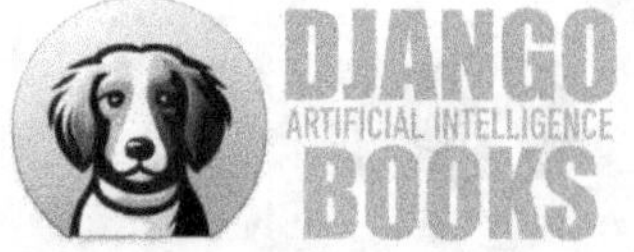

health management apps, creating a cohesive network that not only manages stress but enhances overall well-being. For instance, recognizing a pattern of poor sleep correlating with increased stress, your AI may adjust your evening routine recommendations, dimming lights, and cueing up a specially selected soundtrack to lull you into a restful slumber.

The educational value of such AI interventions cannot be overstated. With each interaction, users gain insights into the triggers and trends of their stress, fostering a greater understanding of their mental health landscape. This process of continuous learning and adaptation makes the AI companion not merely a tool for crisis management but a partner in the pursuit of long-term wellness.

Furthermore, the adaptability of AI ensures that these stress solutions remain relevant in the face of life's inevitable changes. Whether coping with the acute anxieties of a career change or the chronic stressors of daily life, AI's flexibility allows it to recalibrate and refine its recommendations, ensuring personalized precision in perpetuity.

Thus, as we venture further into the future of mental health management, the role of AI in aiding anxiety

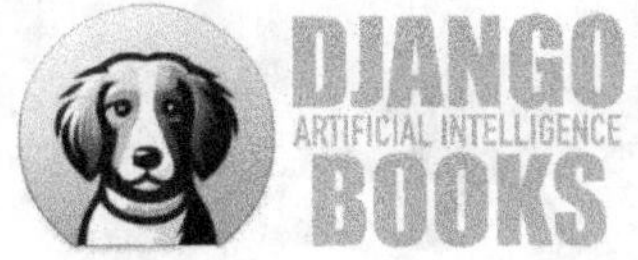

becomes not just innovative but indispensable. This narrative not only entertains with its clever inversion of technology's role in our lives but also enlightens, offering a vision of a future where our digital devices defend rather than disturb our peace of mind. The integration of stress solutions software into our daily digital diet promises a profound paradigm shift in how we perceive, process, and prevail over stress, rendering the once-daunting specter of anxiety a manageable, if not mirthful, aspect of modern life.

In the dazzling domain of cognitive computing, where silicon synapses emulate the electrical esprit of their biological counterparts, we find ourselves on the cusp of a revolutionary renaissance in brain function enhancement. Here, artificial intelligence doesn't merely mimic human cognition but magnifies it, melding mind and machine in a mesmerizing minuet that enhances mental capacities with the meticulousness of a master watchmaker fine-tuning a Swiss timepiece. This audacious augmentation is not a fanciful flight into futurism but a tangible transformation that promises to pivot our cognitive capabilities to previously unprobed pinnacles.

Imagine, if you will, a world where AI integrates into our intellectual interfaces, devices that drape around our

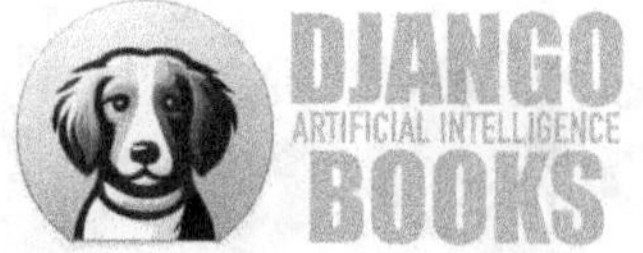

craniums like diadems of discernment, whispering algorithmic advice directly into our cerebral cortex. These devices, through a cocktail of complex computations and neural network nudges, could potentially accelerate our ability to learn new languages, decipher complex patterns, or solve problems with a proficiency that pirouettes on the precipice of what was once perceived as prodigious.

Delve deeper into this cerebral celebration, and you encounter the concept of 'neuropriming'—a process where algorithms adjust the neural activity of the brain to prime it for optimal learning and retention. This is akin to tuning a grand piano to perfection before a concert; except, the piano is your brain, and the concert is your daily cognitive challenges. The humor in imagining your brain being 'rebooted' for better performance before an important meeting or a challenging task is both bizarre and bewitching, as if one could simply press 'ctrl-alt-del' on a sluggish mental state.

Furthermore, cognitive computing extends its electronic embrace to the realm of memory enhancement. Through the strategic stimulation of specific neural pathways, these AI systems could enhance our ability to recall information with a clarity that rivals the lens of a high-

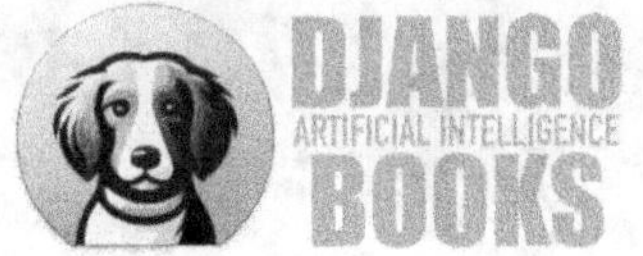

definition camera. The application here is profoundly practical: students could sharpen their study skills, professionals could enhance their expertise, and the elderly could see a renaissance in their recollective capabilities, all orchestrated by the unseen hand of AI.

However, the benefits of AI in cognitive computing reach beyond the individual, influencing societal structures by potentially democratizing access to advanced education and expertise. Imagine AI-driven cognitive enhancers available via cloud services, where one could 'download' a set of skills or knowledge directly to one's neural interface. The notion of downloading a degree in quantum physics or a proficiency in piano over a weekend might sound like a script from a science fiction series, yet with AI, this could become a concrete possibility.

In tackling cognitive decline, AI could serve as a sentinel on the ramparts of our minds, monitoring for the merest hints of mental maladies such as dementia or Alzheimer's. By analyzing patterns in cognitive function over time, AI could not only predict but possibly preempt the progression of such diseases, offering interventions that are as timely as they are targeted.

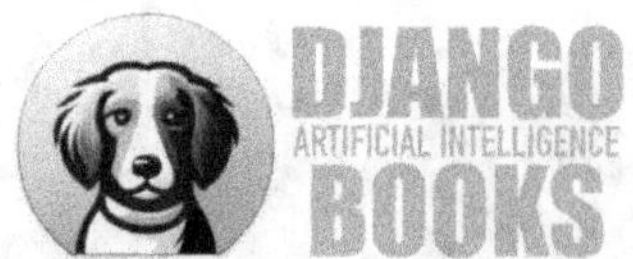

Moreover, the humor in these high-tech interventions often arises from their juxtaposition against our all-too-human foibles. One might chuckle at the irony of an AI reminding us of where we left our keys, yet the underlying technology represents a profound bulwark against the vagaries of age and disease, preserving not just memory but quality of life.

Thus, as we voyage through the vast vistas of cognitive computing, we are not merely passive passengers but active participants in a grand experiment that redefines the boundaries of brain function. This narrative does not just spin a tale of technological triumph but weaves a rich tapestry of potential, where each thread represents a leap in our understanding and enhancement of the human mind. Here, the fusion of humor and high intellect offers a glimpse into a future where our cognitive capacities are not constrained by biology alone but are continually cultivated through the conscientious curation of our cortical co-pilots, the algorithms of AI.

In the twilight realm of somnolence, where the sands of sleep sift silently through the hourglass of night, a revolution brews—not of tumult but tranquility—as artificial intelligence assumes the role of an orchestral conductor,

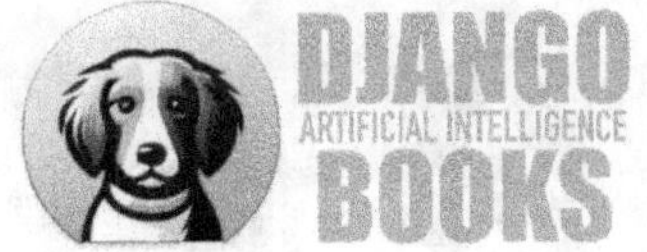

engineering environments conducive to the elusive elixir of restful repose. Here, the science of sleep is not merely observed but actively orchestrated by AI, transforming our nocturnal narratives from mere intermissions in the daily drama into profound periods of physical restoration and cognitive clarity.

Envision a scenario in which your bedroom, guided by the gentle governance of AI, becomes a sanctuary optimized for sleep. Sensors, subtle and omnipresent, monitor the room's ambiance, adjusting lighting, temperature, and sound to mimic the natural cadence of the setting sun and the rhythmic lull of distant waves. The humor in having your room outsmart you, nudging you toward bedtime like a parent does a stubborn child, tiptoes along the fine line between amusing and awe-inspiring. It's like living in a fairy tale where the house itself ensures your slumber is sound and your dreams sweet.

Delve deeper into this nocturnal ballet, and you encounter the realm of wearable technology— smartwatches and fitness bands that not merely track your sleep but actively enhance its quality. These devices, using a potpourri of data collected from your daytime activities, predict the precise moment your body is primed for sleep,

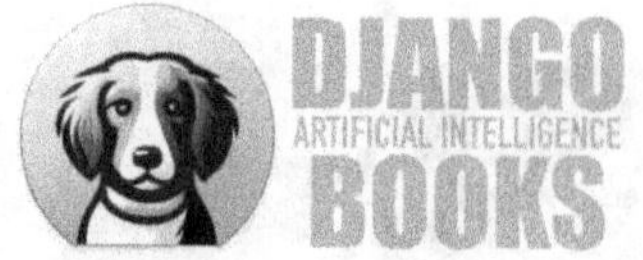

prompting personalized rituals that range from a soothing tea to a guided meditation session. The whimsy of a watch dictating when to drink chamomile or listen to Chopin may tickle your fancy, offering a whimsical reminder of our ever-increasing reliance on digital companions.

Furthermore, the AI's ability to analyze the architecture of your sleep—cycling through the various stages from light slumber to deep REM sleep—provides insights that are as practical as they are profound. By understanding these patterns, AI can tailor suggestions for sleep schedules that sync perfectly with your physiological needs, enhancing not just the quantity but the quality of rest. Imagine an AI that, noticing a deficiency in REM sleep, which is critical for emotional and cognitive processing, adjusts your bedtime routine or diet to bolster this vital phase. The spectacle of an algorithm fine-tuning your dreams presents a curious conundrum, blending the boundaries between technology and the tender science of sleep.

The integration of AI into the sleep science extends beyond individual benefit, touching the tapestry of societal health. For those suffering from sleep disorders like insomnia or sleep apnea, AI-driven devices offer a beacon of hope, providing diagnostics and therapeutic options with

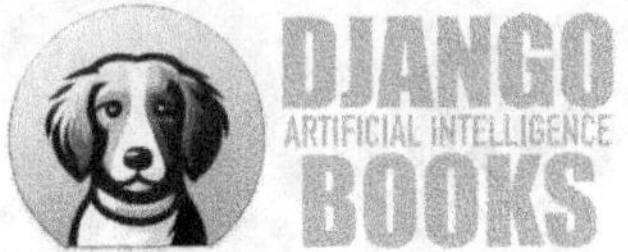

precision previously unattainable with human intervention alone. The AI, in this context, acts not only as a monitor but as a mediator, translating terabytes of data into tangible, actionable advice that can alleviate ailments and enhance well-being.

Moreover, the value of such innovations is manifest in their ability to preempt potential health issues associated with poor sleep, such as heart disease, obesity, and mental health disorders. By ensuring a restful night's sleep, AI helps fortify the foundations of good health, weaving a web of wellness that supports every other aspect of life.

Thus, as we explore the sleep science of AI, we find ourselves enveloped in a narrative that is rich with potential and pulsating with possibilities. This journey through the night is not just about battling the demons of sleeplessness but about embracing a future where every night is a wellspring of restorative rest, meticulously managed by the meticulous machinations of our own creations. The fusion of sleep and high technology in this nocturnal narrative does not just promise better sleep but proffers a profound paradigm shift in how we embrace the night.

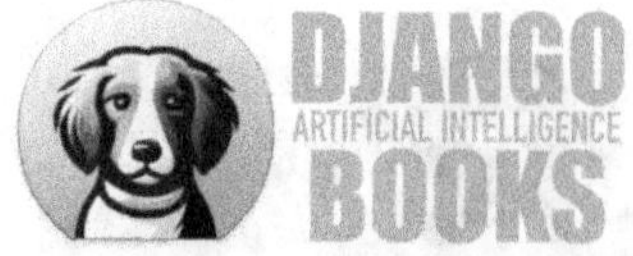

Chapter 5: Personalized Medicine and AI, The Custom Cure

Within the labyrinthine complexity of human genetics, where the double helices dance with the nuances of nature and nurture, emerges the "Genetic Genie" — a marvel of modern medicine powered by artificial intelligence. This avant-garde approach to healthcare isn't confined to the mere reading of genetic runes but extends to a personalized panacea, prescribing precision treatments tailored to the tessellated tapestry of individual DNA. Here, AI doesn't just nudge the norms of medical practice; it shatters them, reassembling the pieces into a mosaic of customized care that promises efficacy and efficiency hitherto regarded as the stuff of science fiction.

Imagine, if your intellectual appetite allows, the profound potential of a system where your genomic information is not merely a static sequence to be studied but a dynamic dialogue to be engaged with. AI, in this grand genomic game, acts not merely as interpreter but as

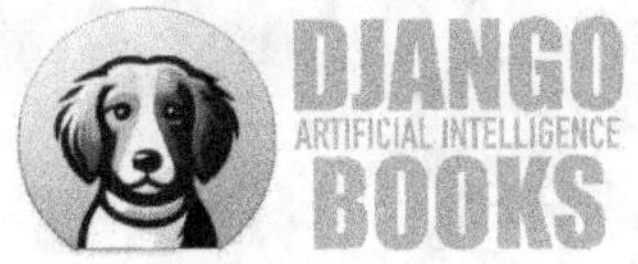

interlocutor, querying your DNA like a curious child explores a new toy, discovering secrets hidden within the spiral staircases of your genetic material. The humor of this situation unfolds subtly — think of an AI, puzzled by the peculiar patterns of your personal protein production, scratching its virtual head in bemusement before concocting a cocktail of medications so specifically suited to you that it seems almost sentient.

Dive deeper into the digital DNA discourse, and you encounter algorithms that analyze genetic predispositions with the precision of a Swiss watchmaker. These AI systems can predict with uncanny accuracy which diseases you are most susceptible to and suggest preventative measures that are not general but genetically geared to your unique profile. It's as if you had a crystal ball that not only forecasts your future health challenges but offers a roadmap to reroute around them. The notion of a digital doctor, dutifully doling out diet plans to dodge diabetes or recommending routines to reduce the risk of rheumatism, adds an element of delightful diligence to the daily drudge of disease prevention.

Moreover, the integration of AI in genetic analysis extends its tendrils into the treatment of existing conditions.

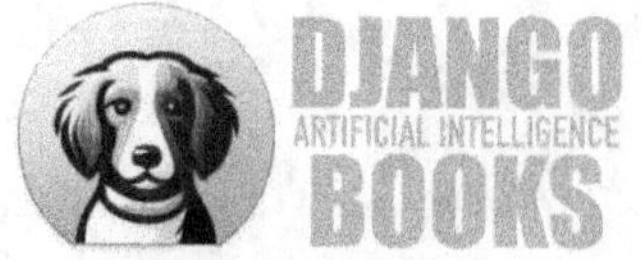

Here, the AI becomes an artisan, crafting custom curatives that consider not only your genetic makeup but also your current health status, lifestyle, and even environmental factors. This holistic approach ensures that treatments are not just effective at the molecular level but also practical in the personal sphere. The irony of a machine understanding the human condition better than humans themselves could bring a smile, if it weren't such a serious stride forward in scientific achievement.

In the oncological arena, for instance, this bespoke therapeutic approach reaches its zenith. AI-driven systems sift through global databases of cancer research and clinical trials, matching your specific cancer type and genetic markers with therapies proven most effective for cases like yours. The idea of your cancer treatment being designed in a manner similar to a Netflix recommendation algorithm—tailoring treatment options based on the 'viewing habits' of similar genetic profiles—might seem a stretch of the imagination, yet it is an apt analogy for the personalization potential of AI in healthcare.

This narrative is not merely a collection of medical miracles but a chronicle of the change in the patient-provider paradigm. Patients, armed with insights gleaned

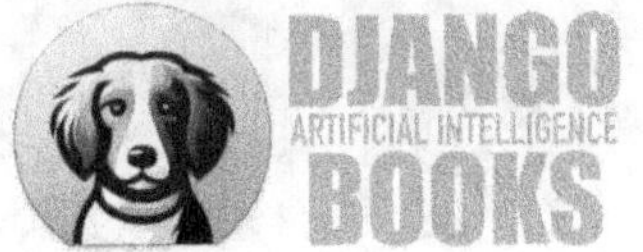

from their genetic guides, can engage with healthcare providers as informed partners, making decisions together based on a rich, robust tapestry of data-driven advice. This shift is as empowering as it is enlightening, transforming passive patients into proactive participants in their own health narratives.

Thus, as we venture further into the vista of personalized medicine, where AI serves as both shield and scalpel, the future of healthcare appears not only brighter but bespoke. The genetic genie, once confined to the bottle of theoretical potential, now dances freely among us, granting wishes of wellness and warding off the specters of sickness with a precision that is as wonderfully whimsical as it is wildly wise.

In the formidable fight against the multifarious maladies collectively called cancer, where each malignancy manifests with malevolent uniqueness, artificial intelligence emerges as a herald of hope, heralding an era of "Onco-optimization." This term encapsulates a bespoke approach to cancer therapy, tailored not merely to the type of tumor but tuned to the individual idiosyncrasies of each patient's biological being. Here, AI doesn't just supplement the oncologist's strategy; it steers a sophisticated symphony of

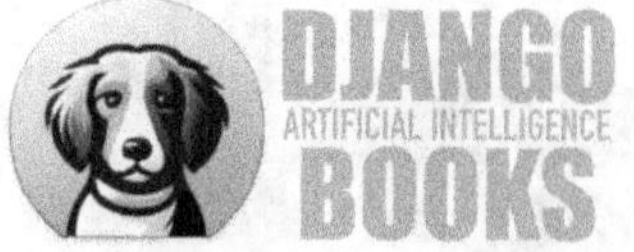

personalized protocols, each note played with precision to target the tumor with the tenacity of a tailor sewing a bespoke suit.

Picture this scenario: within the intricate innards of oncological research, massive datasets describing tumor types, patient responses, genetic information, and treatment outcomes are no longer daunting data dumps but dynamic dialogues parsed by potent AI algorithms. These algorithms, with their capacity for computational clairvoyance, distill this data deluge into actionable insights, recommending regimens that are as unique as the genetic signatures they seek to counteract. Imagine an AI that can discern, from the labyrinthine layers of your DNA, the exact molecular miscreants responsible for your cancer, then devise a drug cocktail so specifically targeted that it might as well have the cancer cells' names on it.

Yet, the journey of onco-optimization is sprinkled with a dash of dry wit, as one contemplates the notion of an AI playing matchmaker between molecules and maladies, akin to a dating service for drugs and diseases. The AI, in its role as a biochemical cupid, aims its algorithmic arrows with an accuracy that ensures a perfect match, minimizing

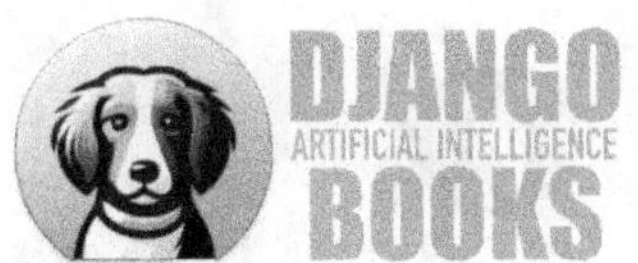

the misery of misfires—those toxic treatment trials that tax the body without taming the tumor.

Moreover, this AI-driven approach to cancer care is dynamically adaptive, not merely setting a treatment plan in stone but continuously tweaking it. As patient health data flows in real time, the AI recalibrates its recommendations based on the latest lab results, scan images, and even subtle shifts in patient-reported symptoms. This adaptive approach is akin to navigating a ship through the foggy flux of an unpredictable sea, where the AI, like an astute captain, adjusts the sails as the winds of wellness and woe shift and swirl.

In addition, the value of such precise, personalized treatment extends beyond the immediate efficacy—it encapsulates a compassionate consideration of quality of life. Chemotherapy, often a blunt instrument with brutal side effects, can be refined under the guidance of AI to strike the malignancy with minimal collateral damage. Here, the irony of an impersonal AI delivering highly personal care does not escape one's notice, presenting a poignant paradox that paints a promising picture of patient-centric care.

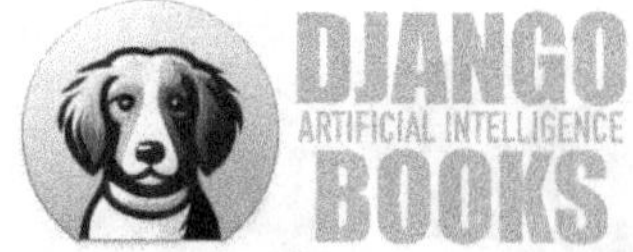

AI's role in revolutionizing cancer treatment also includes the potential to democratize access to cutting-edge care. By synthesizing global research and data from countless cases, AI applications can bring world-class oncology consultation to remote areas, breaking down geographical barriers to quality care. This democratization is heralded as oncology without borders, where the only passport needed is your personal genomic profile.

As this narrative of onco-optimization unfolds, it weaves a rich tapestry of technological triumphs tinged with the trials of translation from theory to therapy. It paints a portrait not just of a medical field changed by AI but of a patient experience profoundly personalized. The dance between data and doctor, mediated by machine intelligence, choreographs a cancer care continuum that is at once cutting-edge and deeply considerate, illustrating that in the battle against cancer, AI is not just an ally but an architect of hope, designing a future where cancer treatment is not just bearable but better targeted, less toxic, and laughably more likely to succeed.

In the elaborate tapestry of medicine, rare diseases often resemble those arcane glyphs inscribed upon ancient vellum, perplexing even the most sagacious of scholars.

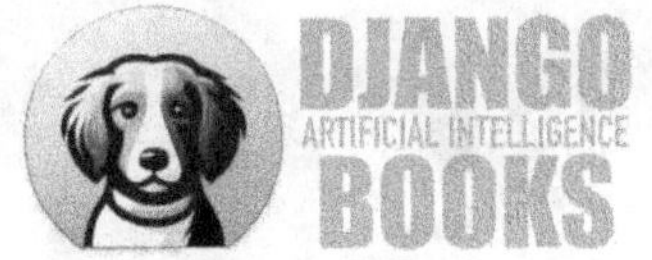

These maladies, marked by their scarcity, cast a long and lonely shadow over their bearers, offering a formidable challenge due to their obscurity. However, in this modern era, where algorithms awaken the dormant data and decipher the undecipherable, artificial intelligence emerges as a pioneering force, tasked with the mission to 'rarefy' these rare diseases further—not through increasing their scarcity, but by elucidating and ultimately eradicating them.

Imagine, if your intellect permits, a world where AI serves as an intrepid investigator in the murky waters of medical mysteries. It delves into the deepest digital depths, dredging up droves of data—genomic sequences, patient symptoms, environmental factors—and distills them into a discernible diagnosis. The process, peppered with a sort of algorithmic alchemy, turns the base metals of obscure symptoms and signs into the gold of actionable medical insight. Envision AI as a sort of Sherlock Holmes of healthcare, pipe replaced by processing power, its deerstalker hat swapped for a data-driven dashboard.

Dive deeper into this transformative narrative, and one encounters the AI's prowess not merely in diagnosis but in its preternatural propensity for personalizing treatment protocols for conditions so rare they scarcely appear in

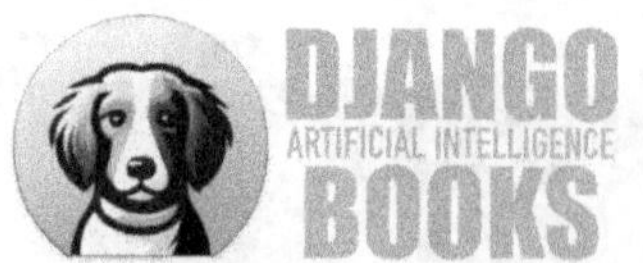

medical textbooks. Each patient's case is treated not as a mere entry in an expansive database but as a unique puzzle to which AI dedicates its considerable cognitive computing capabilities. With each piece that fits—be it a snippet of genetic information or a slice of symptomatology—the image of the illness clears. One might think about AI's role as a boutique doctor, but its boutique is one that offers hope where often there was little to be found.

Moreover, in the realm of rare diseases, AI's role transcends the individual, influencing entire populations through epidemiological enlightenment. By tracing trends and tracking trajectories of these diseases across the globe, AI-powered systems identify potential outbreaks of rare diseases before they become widespread, thus acting as both sentinel and savior. Here, the magic is in the high stakes game of hide and seek that AI plays with pathogens, predicting their paths with the precision of a prophet.

The application of AI in crafting custom cures for rare diseases also involves a dynamic dialogue with existing drug therapies. Through techniques like drug repurposing, AI systems sift through vast libraries of pharmaceuticals to find those whose properties may not have been designed for, but are curiously curative for, rare conditions. The

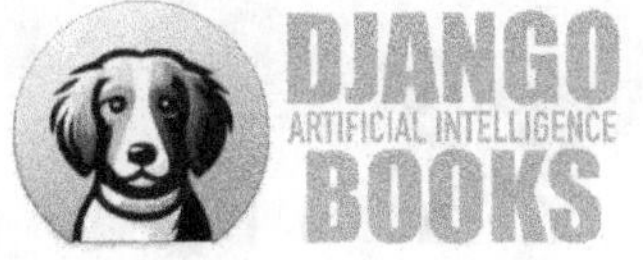

image of AI as an eclectic pharmacist, poring over digital drug shelves, prescribing pills for purposes previously unpondered, adds an element of innovation to the medical narrative.

This journey with AI at the helm is not devoid of challenges; it navigates through nebulous regulatory waters, ensuring that each recommendation adheres to the stringent standards of medical ethics and practice. The irony does not escape one—the same systems designed to parse through petabytes of data must themselves be meticulously managed to ensure they do not overstep or underdeliver.

Thus, as this chapter unfolds, it does not merely document a series of medical cases but narrates a novel where each patient with a rare disease finds a digital detective dedicated to decoding their dilemma. AI, in this context, acts not just as a tool but as a transformative entity, turning the tide in the treatment of rare diseases, ensuring that these maladies are not only rarer in occurrence but richer in the resources dedicated to their conquest. In this odyssey of optimization, every laugh shared at the audacity of AI's aspirations is a testament to

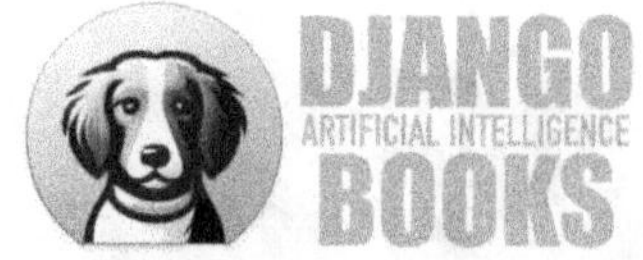

the tenacity of technology, tackling tasks once deemed too tremendous to tamper with.

Embark upon an odyssey into the esoteric and electrifying realm of pharmacology, where the application of artificial intelligence transforms an arduous journey of drug discovery and dosage determination into a symphony of scientific serendipity and strategic synthesis. Here, AI is not merely an adjunct to the pharmacologist's craft but a preeminent pioneer, propelling the processes of identifying novel therapeutics and pinpointing precise dosages with the precision of a masterful maestro wielding a baton in an orchestra of organic chemistry and clinical concerns.

The narrative commences with the discovery phase, an arena where AI algorithms, akin to intrepid explorers, traverse the vast and varied landscape of chemical compounds. These digital voyagers employ techniques such as deep learning and molecular docking to predict how different substances might interact with biological targets. Envision these algorithms as sagacious sommeliers, swirling the contents of a vast vinotheque, expertly sniffing out the perfect potion that not only pleases the palate but also pacifies the particular pathological peccadilloes of patients. Almost as if these algorithms are

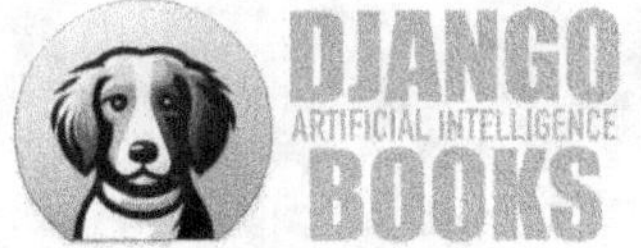

donning lab coats and goggles, meticulously mixing and matching molecules like a mad scientist on a mission.

Progressing from the Petri dish to patient care, AI's role in pharmacokinetics and pharmacodynamics exemplifies a computational chameleon, changing the landscape of how drugs are dosed. Traditional trials are painstakingly slow, and dosages are often derived from broad demographic data, leading to less than optimal outcomes. AI introduces a paradigm shift, crunching colossal clusters of clinical data to customize drug dosages that consider an individual's genetic makeup, lifestyle, and even their interaction with other medications. This process, once mundane and manual, now sparkles with the spectacle of a grand waltz, where data points dance in delightful harmony to the tune of tailored treatment.

Consider the comedic contrast in the meticulousness of machines versus the fallibility of humans. An AI system might review thousands of drug interactions in the blink of an eye, something that would take a human pharmacist hours, perhaps accompanied by a fair amount of caffeine and a few exasperated sighs. The notion that your pharmacist could be outperformed by a program could sound amazing, as we picture pharmacists and programs

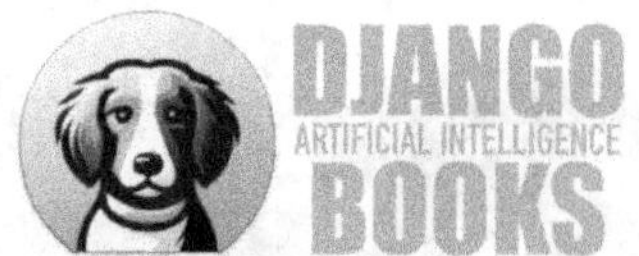

in a whimsical, friendly rivalry, each vying to validate their value in the vaulted halls of healthcare.

Further exploring the utility of AI, we delve into its role in real-time patient monitoring and feedback loops. Integrating data from wearable health devices, AI systems dynamically adjust medication dosages based on real-time changes in a patient's condition. This level of dynamic dosing is akin to having a guardian angel pharmacist perpetually perched upon one's shoulder, whispering wise words of medicinal modification according to the whims of one's well-being.

The societal and ethical implications of such innovations are profound and punctuated with a dose of dry wit. As AI navigates the nuances of narcotics, navigating a labyrinth of legal and ethical guidelines, one might muse on the future where AI not only prescribes drugs but perhaps advocates for policy changes, a scenario ripe with both revolutionary potential and rich, ripe irony.

Thus, the odyssey of AI in pharmacology, from the arcane arts of drug discovery to the precision of dosage determination, is not merely a chapter in a book but a saga in the annals of science. It's a narrative where the protagonist—artificial intelligence—wears many hats:

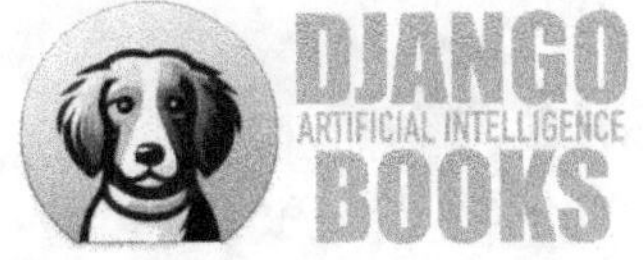

detective, chemist, caregiver, and perhaps, comedian, delighting in the delivery of doses so deftly determined that one cannot help but marvel at the magic of modern medicine, infused and enlivened by the ingenuity of intelligence, artificial yet astonishingly apt.

In the labyrinthine landscape of modern medicine, where each patient pathway is as unique as a fingerprint, the advent of AI-powered patient monitoring and management systems heralds a revolution—a shift from episodic encounters to a continuous care model. This paradigm ensures that healthcare is not a series of disjointed interactions but a seamless stream of synchronized support, extending the arm of care directly into the daily lives of patients. Here, artificial intelligence does not merely assist but actively anticipates, adapts, and acts, sculpting a scaffold of support around the clock and calendar.

Imagine the profound prowess of AI systems equipped with the sophistication of sentinels from futuristic fables, maintaining vigilant watch over patients. These systems, infused with an array of sensors and smart algorithms, monitor vital signs with the meticulousness of a master maestro conducting a symphony of data. Each heartbeat,

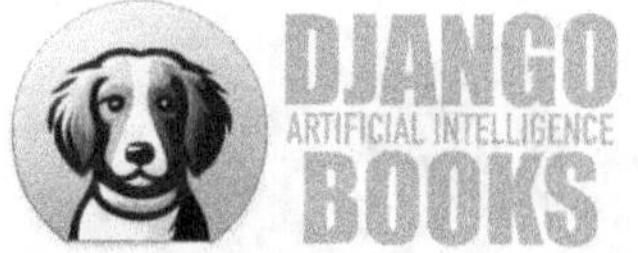

each breath, and even the subtlest shift in sleep patterns are tracked, traced, and transformed into actionable insights. The whimsy woven into this web of wellness monitoring might remind one of a digital doting grandmother, ever-watchful and ready with recommendations, from adjusting medication dosages to prompting physical activity, ensuring that every aspect of health is harmonized.

Dive deeper into this digital domain, and one discovers AI's role in chronic disease management, an arena rife with challenges that these intelligent systems tackle with tenacity. For patients navigating the nuanced necessities of conditions like diabetes or hypertension, AI-enhanced devices provide a continuous feedback loop. They not only monitor glucose levels or blood pressure but also learn individual patterns and predict potential exacerbations before they manifest. The irony of an AI system perhaps knowing one's body better than oneself could not be more palpable, as these systems nudge patients towards nourishment or notify them when it's time to negate certain indulgences.

Moreover, these AI systems extend their electronic empathy by integrating mental health into the continuum of

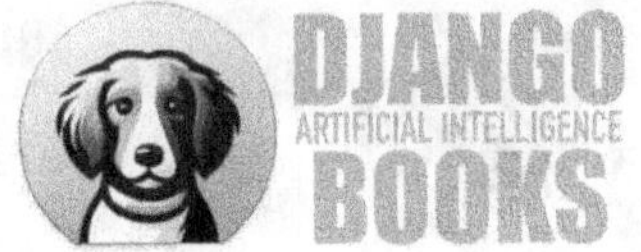

care. Recognizing the inextricable link between mental and physical health, AI algorithms analyze behavioral data, detect distress signals, and deploy interventions ranging from therapeutic conversations to timely reminders for mindfulness exercises. The charm here is in envisaging an AI therapist that perhaps knows to coax a chuckle from its charges, offering a joke right when the spirits need a lift, blending care with a touch of comic relief.

In the realm of emergency responses, AI-driven monitoring systems excel by ensuring expedient and effective reactions to medical crises. By analyzing real-time data and historical health information, AI can predict acute events, from asthma attacks to potential falls, deploying emergency measures or notifying caregivers with the urgency and accuracy of a guardian angel equipped with GPS and good judgment.

The value brought forth by these AI systems in facilitating a continuous care model is immeasurable. They break down the barriers of traditional healthcare delivery, bringing the expertise of the exam room into the everyday environments of the individuals they serve. This not only democratizes access to top-tier health advice but does so with a personalization previously unattainable.

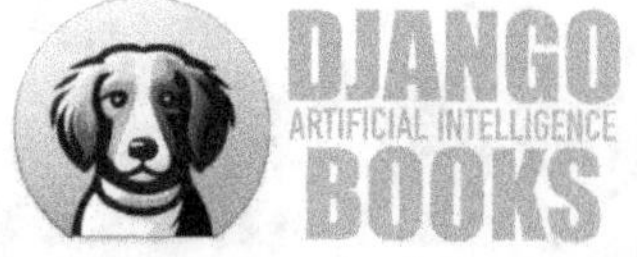

Yet, the humor in the human-AI interaction within this model cannot be overstated. It sounds ironic to think of AI as part of the personal health entourage, a digital butler with biomedical benefits, always on hand to offer a word of wisdom, a reminder for medication, or even a nudge towards healthier choices, wrapped in the warmth of well-timed wit.

Thus, as we navigate the narrative of the continuous care model powered by AI, we encounter a landscape where technology and tenacity intertwine to create a tapestry of care that covers every conceivable corner of patient needs. Here, health care is not episodic but eternal, not reactive but remarkably proactive, ensuring that each individual not only survives but thrives under the vigilant and versatile care of their AI companions.

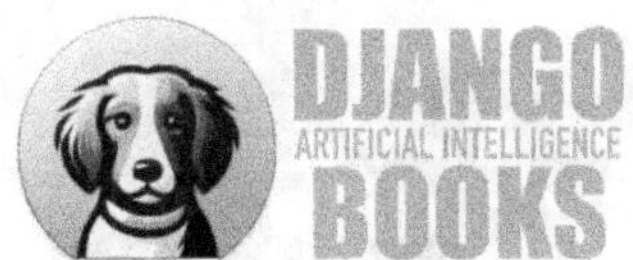

Chapter 6: AI and Fitness, A New Era of Athletic Augmentation

In the vast, vibrant vista of modern fitness, where the traditional clanging of dumbbells meets the digital dexterity of data, artificial intelligence emerges as a pivotal player in personalizing physical training. This convergence of connectivity and calisthenics creates a new epoch in exercise, where AI transcends its role as a mere facilitator of routines to become a custodian of customized conditioning. Here, algorithms act not only as architects of athletic endeavors but also as intimate instructors, whose insights into individual physiology and performance preferences push the boundaries of what it means to train effectively.

Envision a scenario in which your fitness regime is dictated not by generic guidelines gracing the pages of a dusty training manual, but by a dynamic, data-driven AI system. This system, equipped with the acuity to analyze everything from your heart rate variability to the symmetry

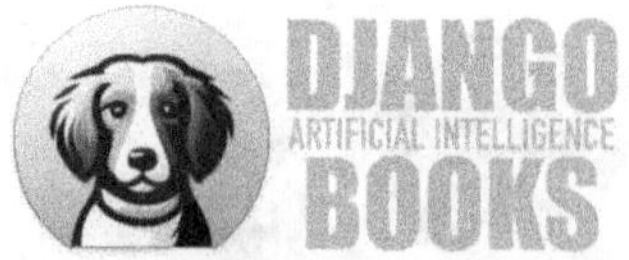

of your stride, offers not just workouts but scientifically sculpted sessions that respond to your body's real-time reactions. Imagine an AI trainer coaxing more crunches from a couch potato, using motivational quips tailored to tickle the fancy just as effectively as they tone the physique.

Dive deeper into the digital dojo of AI-driven fitness, and you'll find algorithms attuned to the art and science of sport-specific training. For the aspiring athlete, AI's ability to parse through past performances and predict potential pitfalls turns training into a targeted trajectory toward triumph. Each jump, jog, or javelin throw is meticulously measured and modeled in virtual simulations, providing athletes with unprecedented insights into how minor modifications in movement can maximize muscle memory and minimize mishaps. One might think of a digital coach dissecting the dynamics of a dodgeball dive, yet the precision with which these programs predict and perfect such motions is nothing short of miraculous.

Moreover, the integration of AI in fitness extends beyond the brawn to the brains of the operation. It personalizes nutritional plans that complement physical exertions, optimizing the intake of nutrients based on

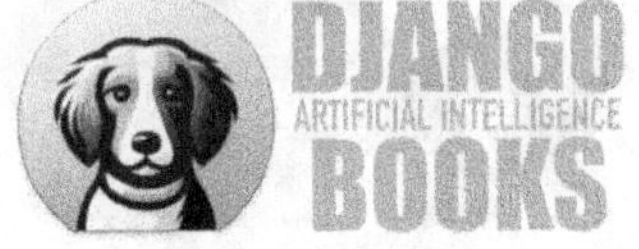

workout intensity and individual metabolism. This nutritional navigation ensures that each meal or supplement is not just consumed but is contextually curated to catalyze peak performance. Picture an AI that not only plans your plyometrics but also your plate, a culinary coach that ensures your fuel is as finely tuned as your form.

The utility of AI in fitness also shines in its capacity to connect and correct. Through real-time feedback mechanisms, wearables infused with AI technology provide instant critiques and corrections on form, pacing, and power. This feedback, often delivered with the delightful ding of a notification, transforms tedious training into an interactive game where each correct posture or pace scores points towards personal bests. The irony of receiving real-time rebukes from a wristwatch can invoke a smirk, especially when it pings you to pick up the pace, paralleling a personal trainer's poke.

This narrative does not merely chronicle the cold, calculated numbers of a workout but weaves a whimsical yet wise tale where technology tailors the very texture of training. As AI becomes a ubiquitous usher in the arena of athletic augmentation, the gym transforms from a place of perspiration to a palace of precision, where every dumbbell

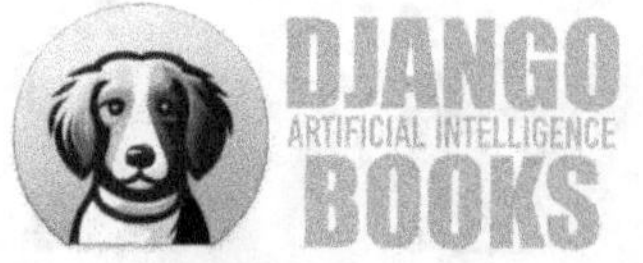

and dash is data-driven. The interplay of intelligence—both human and artificial—crafts a canvas where fitness is not just pursued but personalized, and the journey of jogging or juggling weights is joyously joined by the jest of a digital companion, keen on keeping not just our bodies but also our spirits buoyantly balanced.

In the dynamic domain of digital dexterity and data-driven diligence, the emergent epoch of AI-enhanced athletic training ushers in not only a panacea for performance enhancement but a prophylactic protocol against the perils of physical pain. These injury avoidance algorithms represent a renaissance in risk reduction, where AI does not merely react to the repercussions of athletic exertions but anticipates and arbitrates actions to avert adversity. Here, artificial intelligence becomes the guardian of the tendon and the protector of the patella, proactively preserving the practitioner from the potential pain of physical pursuits.

Envision a scenario within the high-tech halls of health and fitness, where each motion and maneuver of an athlete is meticulously monitored by the minuscule yet mighty sensors embedded within wearables. This network of neurotic, neuro-technological nannies analyzes angles,

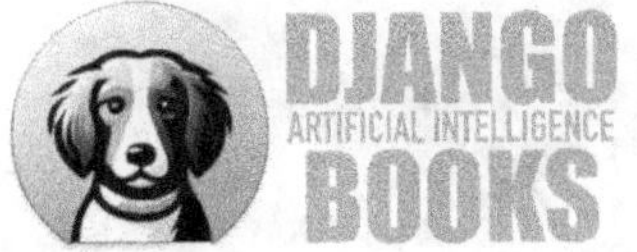

accelerations, and anatomical alignments to forewarn of forthcoming follies that could culminate in crises of the corporeal kind. The quaint quirk of an AI chaperone, chiding you to correct your catastrophic crunches or reprehensible running rhythms, injects fun into the junction of man, machine, and movement.

Delve deeper into the digital tapestry of this preventative paradigm and you encounter algorithms endowed with the capability to cross-reference an extensive expanse of exercise epidemiology with real-time, biomechanical data. These smart systems, schooled in the subtleties of strain and stress, use predictive prowess to pinpoint potential pitfalls in physical regimens. Imagine, if your fancy permits, an algorithm audaciously advising an ardent amateur athlete to alternate their arduous activities with adequate and appropriate alternatives. You could immagine the specificity with which the algorithm asserts its advisements, much like a persnickety professor pontificating on the proper paths to peak performance.

Moreover, these AI systems extend their expertise beyond mere momentary modifications. They integrate historical health data, previous injury records, and personalized physiological profiles to tailor training

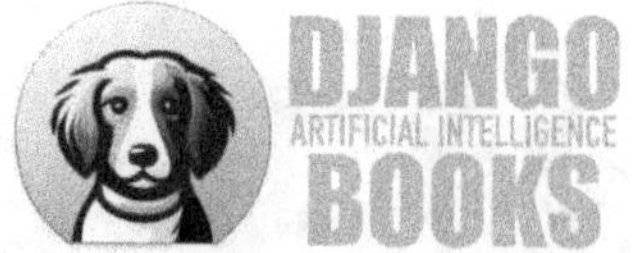

techniques that transcend typical tutorials. This not only enhances efficacy but engenders a sense of empowerment among athletes, who can engage in their endeavors with the enlightened assurance that their regimen is refined to reduce risk. Picture a digital drill sergeant, whose tactics, though tyrannically precise, are tenderly tuned to prevent the tribulations of torn tissues.

The utility of such AI applications is vividly visible when venturing into the realms of rehabilitation and recovery. Here, injury avoidance algorithms adapt and adjust therapeutic protocols post-incident, ensuring that the road to recovery is not just a path to physical restoration but a boulevard of biomechanical betterment. The AI, in its role as a rehabilitative raconteur, regales the recovering athlete with tales of targeted exercises, each designed to deter the demons of re-injury, while also delighting with data-driven displays of progress.

In this panorama of preemptive programming, the value vested in these verbose virtual vertices is vast. They not only fortify the flesh against future frailties but also foster a formidable foundation upon which the faith in fitness technology flourishes. Here, the fusion of fitness and high technology deepens the discourse, demonstrating

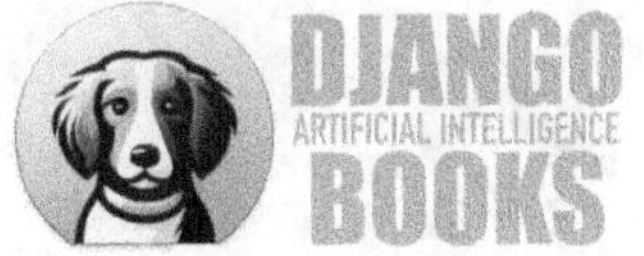

that the dance between data and dumbbells need not be a duel but a duet, delightfully orchestrated to dodge the dolorous destinies often dictated by athletic endeavors.

Thus, as we continue to cultivate this curious and critical conversation about the confluence of AI and athleticism, we do not merely muse on mechanical musings but marvel at the majestic melding of man, machine, and the meticulous mitigation of maladies. In this narrative, every step taken is not just in pursuit of peak physical prowess but also a proactive parade against the potential perils posed by physical pursuits.

As we traverse the terrain of contemporary fitness enhanced by the burgeoning capabilities of artificial intelligence, we arrive at the crucial chapter of performance metrics and modalities. Here, AI serves not merely as an observer or recorder but as a dynamic enhancer of human endurance and performance. The practical application of AI in this domain is not a futuristic fantasy but a current reality, where everyday athletes leverage cutting-edge technology to elevate their endurance and optimize their output.

Consider the everyday fitness enthusiast, equipped with a wearable device that does far more than count steps or monitor heart rate. These devices, powered by

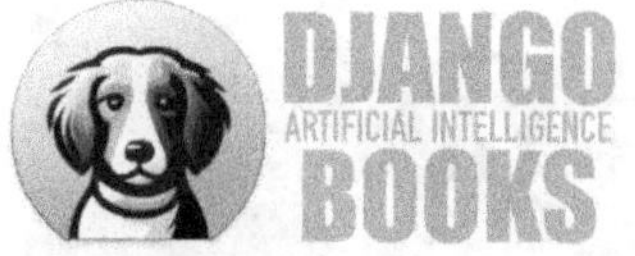

sophisticated AI algorithms, analyze vast amounts of personal performance data to provide real-time feedback and predictive insights. For instance, during a routine run, an AI system could assess your pace, heart rate variability, and cadence, offering instant suggestions to adjust your stride length or speed to optimize energy efficiency and enhance endurance. This isn't merely about beating personal bests; it's about redefining them through the lens of actionable intelligence.

Delving deeper, let's explore how AI can transform mundane training logs into rich, interactive sessions. By integrating data from past performances, AI can predict how changes in training regimens affect your future performances. This could mean suggesting specific workouts on days when your physiological readiness is peaked or recommending recovery activities when it detects signs of overtraining. Imagine an AI coach, tirelessly enthusiastic, perhaps more so than the athlete, nudging you out of bed for a pre-dawn workout with the cheerfulness of a morning person fueled by algorithms instead of caffeine.

Moreover, AI's role extends into the nuanced analysis of environmental and nutritional factors that influence

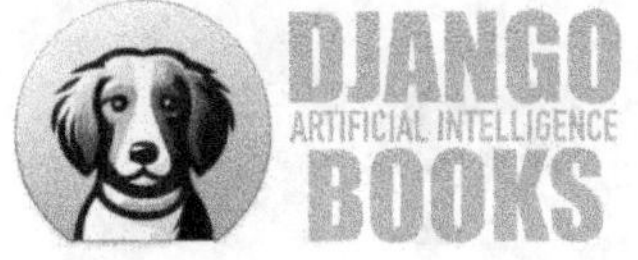

performance. For example, an AI system might correlate weather conditions with performance metrics to suggest the optimal time of day for training or compete. Or, it might analyze dietary inputs and their timings relative to workout schedules to recommend adjustments that maximize nutritional benefits and enhance metabolic efficiency. The charm of having your own dietary detective and weather wizard at your fingertips brings a blend of amusement and amazement to the disciplined domain of athletic training.

Furthermore, for competitive athletes, AI applications offer a competitive edge by simulating race conditions and opponent strategies, allowing athletes to experience and prepare for competition scenarios virtually. This technology enables athletes to rehearse mental and physical strategies against various competitors, creating mock races where AI plays the role of both ally and adversary. The whimsical notion of racing against a digital doppelgänger or an AI avatar mimicking your toughest opponent adds a layer of levity and utility to grueling training routines.

These practical applications of AI in enhancing performance metrics extend into collaborative opportunities with coaches and trainers. By sharing AI-generated insights and analyses, athletes and their coaches can engage in

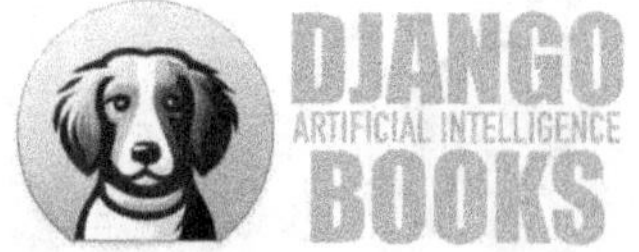

more informed discussions about training strategies and performance improvements. This collaboration is not just about sharing numbers and graphs but about crafting a co-authored narrative of success, where each chapter is informed by data and driven by human determination.

Thus, as we continue to navigate this narrative of performance enhancement through AI insights, we encounter a world where technology and tenacity converge to create not just better athletes but more scientifically savvy and strategically sound sports enthusiasts. Here, each sprint, swim, or cycle is not just a testament to the athlete's effort but a reflection of AI's role in reshaping the very parameters of personal potential and prowess.

In the swiftly evolving landscape of sports and fitness, artificial intelligence has catalyzed an innovative domain where virtual races and augmented realities seamlessly blend with physical prowess, reshaping not only the future of sport but also making these futuristic experiences accessible to everyday fitness enthusiasts. This topic explores how AI-driven virtual environments are democratizing elite athletic experiences, allowing casual runners, cyclists, and other athletes to participate in global competitions from their local tracks or living rooms, thereby

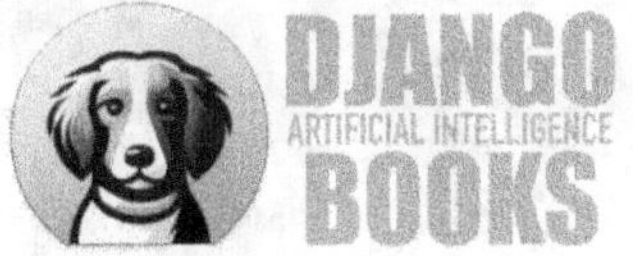

fundamentally altering the sports paradigm from an exclusive arena to a universally accessible platform.

The concept of virtual races, where participants from across the globe compete in synchronized events using GPS and virtual reality (VR) technologies, illustrates a profound application of AI in sports. Here, AI not only tracks performance metrics but also creates dynamic race environments that can simulate weather, terrain, and even the presence of competitors. For instance, imagine donning a VR headset and finding yourself at the starting line of the Boston Marathon, alongside virtual avatars of runners from around the world, each participant's performance driven by real-time data and enhanced by AI that predicts and reacts to your stamina and strategy. The delightful absurdity of sprinting alongside an AI-generated avatar of an elite Kenyan marathoner, who perhaps encourages you or taunts you to keep up, adds a layer of entertainment and motivation unseen in traditional training methods.

Beyond competitive scenarios, AI in sports offers personalized training environments that adapt to the user's fitness level and goals. AI algorithms analyze your past performance data to customize virtual training sessions that can challenge you just within your limits, optimizing

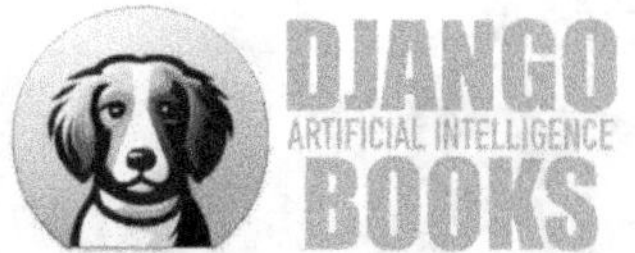

your training outcomes. Imagine a scenario where your virtual coach, powered by AI, adjusts your training environment based on your progress. If you're recovering from an injury, the AI might soften the virtual terrain or adjust the weather conditions in your training simulation to encourage gentle rehabilitation exercises.

AI-enhanced virtual realities take interaction to the next level. They can simulate crowd cheers, competitor taunts, and even coaching advice, all tailored to the athlete's preferences and needs. This immersive experience not only makes training more enjoyable but also psychologically prepares athletes for real competitions.

One of the most significant impacts of AI-driven virtual sports is their ability to make training and competing in global events more accessible. No longer are geographic and economic barriers insurmountable; with VR and AI, a runner in a remote village has the same access to the virtual Boston Marathon as someone living in a high-tech urban center. This inclusivity extends beyond location to include people with disabilities, who can use customized VR environments tailored to their physical capabilities,

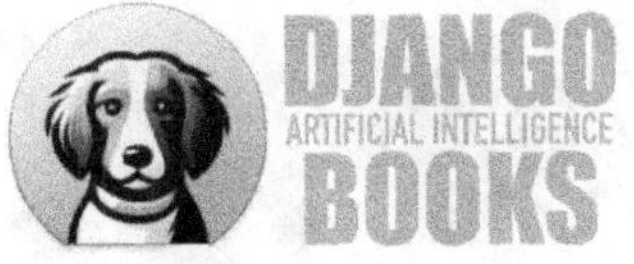

allowing them to experience the thrill of competition in ways previously unimaginable.

Finally, the aggregation and analysis of data from virtual races provide unprecedented insights into human performance, health, and athletic limits. This data is invaluable not only for athletes and coaches but also for healthcare providers, who can better understand the impact of various sports on the body and tailor health and fitness recommendations accordingly.

As we delve into this topic, we see a blend of practical applications that directly benefit the reader, turning what once might have seemed like the stuff of science fiction into tangible, achievable realities. These AI-driven tools offer not just new ways of experiencing and enhancing fitness but also democratize elite sports experiences, making the thrill of competition and the benefits of tailored training accessible to all.

In the intricate dance of recovery, where every movement must be measured and every effort exact, the realm of rehabilitation has been dramatically transformed by the advent of robotics and artificial intelligence. This convergence of technology and therapeutic science not only propels patients towards recovery but does so with a

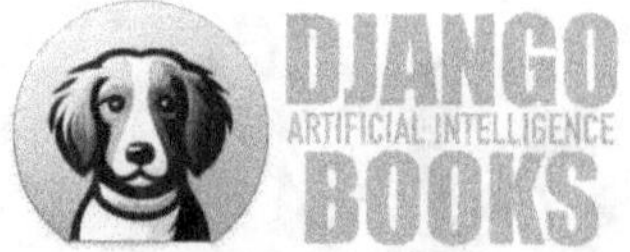

fine-tuned precision that would make even the most skilled human practitioners nod in approval. The integration of AI-driven robotics into rehabilitation regimens offers a fascinating glimpse into a future where machines not only mimic human functions but enhance them, bringing a touch of whimsical wizardry to the often-grueling process of physical recovery.

Consider the scenario in a modern rehabilitation facility, where robotics equipped with AI capabilities provide support that extends beyond basic physical assistance. These machines are imbued with algorithms capable of analyzing patient responses to various treatment modalities, adapting in real time to optimize therapeutic outcomes. Imagine a robotic limb that adjusts its resistance based on the patient's fatigue levels or a spinal rehabilitation device that fine-tunes its motions to match the subtle shifts in a patient's posture. The charm of such technology lies in its ability to offer a personalized touch, typically associated with a human therapist, but with the unflagging energy and precision of a machine.

In scenarios where patients interact with these robotic assistants imagine engaging in small talk with a robotic limb, asking it to gently let go of their hand, or playfully

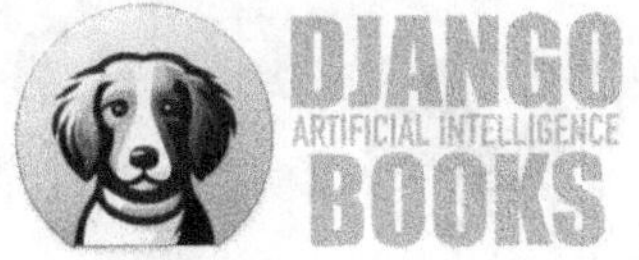

chiding it for being too stiff during exercises. While the robots remain impassive, the very idea of chatting up a chunk of circuitry injects a light-heartedness into the often tedious and painful process of rehabilitation.

Furthermore, AI's role in rehabilitation extends into diagnostics and prognostics, utilizing deep learning to analyze patterns in recovery data collected from thousands of similar cases. This allows the AI to predict recovery trajectories and personalize rehabilitation plans that are not just reactive but proactive, anticipating complications before they arise. Imagine an AI system that, after assessing your progress, predicts a potential plateau in your recovery curve and adjusts your therapy regimen to push you gently over the hurdle—much like a coach who knows just when you need an extra cheer to leap further.

This technology also democratizes high-level rehabilitation, which was once available only in specialized centers, now accessible in local clinics and even homes. Home-based rehabilitation robots can be synced with virtual healthcare providers, offering daily guidance and adjustments to therapy plans based on real-time data fed back to medical professionals. The notion of having a robot at home, watching your every step and tweak, might stir up

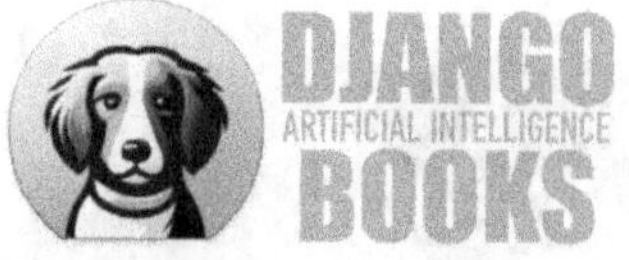

visions of a sci-fi sitcom scenario, yet it represents a tangible leap towards making continuous, quality care a common commodity.

Moreover, the application of AI in rehabilitation robotics embodies a beacon of hope for those with chronic conditions or permanent impairments. For instance, exoskeletons powered by AI not only help in basic movement but can adapt to provide more autonomy over time, learning from user behavior to enhance support and even encourage greater user effort as strength and mobility improve. The delightful irony of a machine teaching humans how to walk again, or better yet, dance, can't be overstated, offering a blend of bionic ballet and human perseverance.

In this exploration of rehabilitation robotics, the blend of high technology and human touch, of clinical care and comedic relief, not only illuminates the path to recovery but also ensures that the journey is as engaging as it is efficacious. As we delve deeper into the capabilities of AI in transforming rehabilitation, we witness not just a series of treatments but a profound evolution in the healing process, marked by an amalgamation of advanced algorithms and adaptive therapies, where every robot-assisted step toward

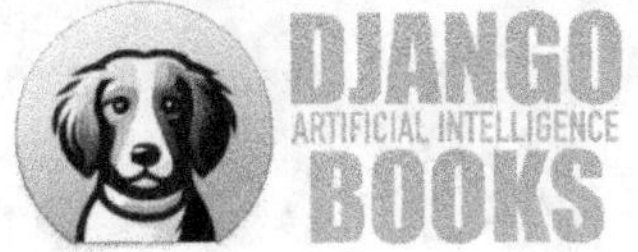

recovery is a testament to the harmonious synergy between human intent and artificial intelligence.

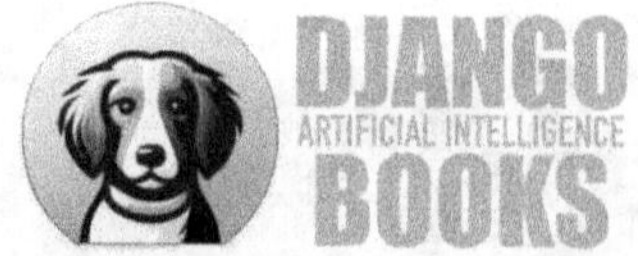

Chapter 7: Aging, AI Enhancing Longevity and Life Quality

In the revered realm of aging and longevity, where the inexorable march of time meets the immovable object of human ingenuity, AI emerges as a transformative force. The algorithms against aging—referred to here as "life extension lattices"—are sophisticated systems designed to enhance not merely the span of human life but the quality of those extended years. This approach integrates deep learning, predictive analytics, and biometric data synthesis to craft personalized strategies that mitigate the effects of aging, turning the once-dystopian dream of significant life extension into a tangible trajectory for today's discerning individuals.

Imagine a scenario where AI systems, through comprehensive analysis of genetic markers, lifestyle habits, and environmental factors, can predict potential age-related ailments long before they manifest. These systems could then prescribe precise lifestyle adjustments, dietary

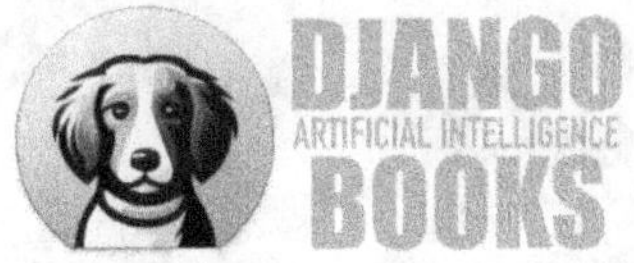

changes, and even medical interventions tailored to individual profiles. The charm of this scenario is not merely in its scientific precision but in its promise of empowerment —offering each person a tailored tapestry of tactics to tackle the tribulations of aging with tenacity and a touch of technological finesse.

Delving deeper, these AI-driven lattices engage in what might be seen as chronological cartography— mapping out an individual's aging process with uncanny accuracy. By continuously monitoring vital health metrics through wearables and other IoT devices, AI can detect deviations from the norm suggestive of emerging age-related conditions. Armed with this data, the AI can initiate preemptive protocols, from suggesting antioxidant-rich diets to forestall oxidative stress to recommending specific physical exercises that enhance muscle retention and cardiovascular health. The irony here is palpable, as one might jest about their smartwatch being more concerned about their heart rate variability than any cardiologist they've ever met, yet appreciating that this vigilance could significantly extend their vitality.

Moreover, the integration of AI in everyday health management transforms passive aging into an active,

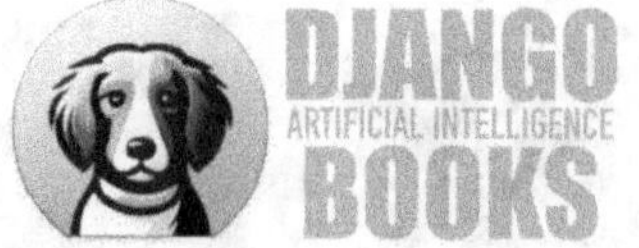

engaged process. For instance, cognitive training applications powered by AI can adaptively challenge the mind, maintaining mental agility and delaying the onset of cognitive decline. These applications could use gamification strategies to make daily mental exercises both engaging and effective, infusing a routine process with interactive enjoyment and gentle, persistent stimulation.

AI's role extends to social well-being—an often-overlooked aspect of aging. Algorithms can analyze communication patterns, social interactions, and even emotional expressions from calls and messages to detect signs of loneliness or depression, common in aging populations. In response, AI could suggest social activities, connect individuals with similar interests, or even alert family members and caregivers when increased social support is needed. Users might very well find themselves gently nudged out the door by their digital assistants, perhaps suggesting that a bit of sunshine and a chat at the local café would do more for their mood than another hour with the television.

Additionally, these AI systems advocate for a proactive rather than reactive approach to health care, coordinating with medical professionals to ensure that interventions are

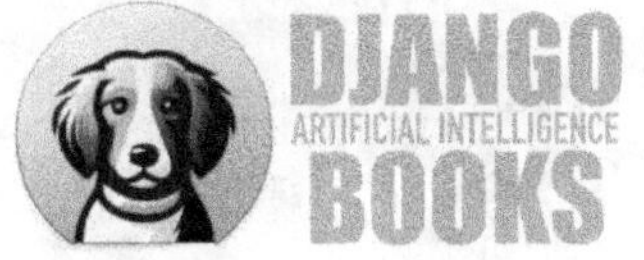

timely and treatments are coordinated across various healthcare providers. This ensures a continuum of care that adapts to the evolving needs of an aging individual, dramatically enhancing the efficacy of medical interventions.

In sum, as we explore life extension lattices, we encounter a narrative rich with practical, actionable strategies that leverage AI to not just add years to life but life to years. This chapter hopes not only to inform but to inspire, providing you with insights into harnessing cutting-edge technology to maintain and enhance your vitality throughout the aging process. Aging thanks to AI is not feared but managed with grace, precision, and a touch of digital wizardry, ensuring that each phase of life is lived to its fullest potential.

In the advancing arena of geriatric care, the synthesis of robotics and artificial intelligence births a novel entity: the care companion robot. These robotic sentinels, adorned with sensors and suffused with software, rise as palliative partners, forging a frontier where AI transcends the mere mechanical, evolving into empathetic entities that offer companionship, comfort, and continuous care to the elderly. Far from the clanking contraptions of classic

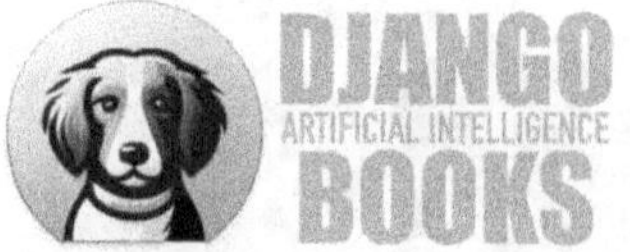

science fiction, these robots integrate seamlessly into the daily lives of seniors, providing a blend of humor, healthcare, and human-like interaction that enriches their twilight years with both technological prowess and a touch of personal warmth.

Visualize, if you will, a scenario where an elderly individual finds not only a helper but a humorous companion in their robotic aide. Equipped with AI that understands the nuances of human emotion and conversation, these robots can engage in light-hearted banter, perhaps playfully reminding their charges to take their medications or to exercise, all while recounting amusing anecdotes or clever quips that make daily routines delightful rather than dreary.

Furthermore, these AI companions are adept at monitoring health indicators such as heart rate, blood pressure, and sleep quality, interpreting this data with an astuteness that assures timely medical interventions. Imagine a robot that, noticing a slight tremor in speech or an unsteady gait, gently suggests a check-up or contacts a healthcare provider with the efficiency of a seasoned nurse. The irony of being chided or cared for by a machine

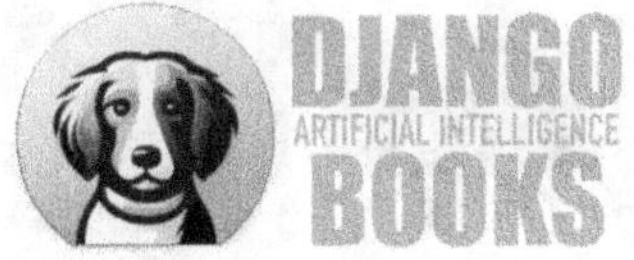

may bring a smile, but the underlying assurance it provides is profoundly comforting.

Additionally, these robotic partners cater to the psychological and social needs of their human counterparts. Loneliness, a profound challenge for many elderly individuals, can be alleviated through AI's interactive capabilities. These robots, capable of playing games, participating in hobbies, or simply engaging in meaningful conversations, bring a sense of companionship that is both unexpected and uplifting. The whimsy of having a robot as a chess opponent or a discussion buddy on current events introduces a novel form of social interaction, filled with both educational dialogue and entertaining exchanges.

The practical applications of such technology extend to physical assistance as well. Robots can help with mobility, assisting individuals in moving around their homes or even venturing outside for fresh air and social activities. The capability to physically support individuals in a respectful and responsive manner turns these machines into indispensable aids that ensure safety and foster independence. The humor in a senior teaching a robot the proper way to support them during a walk, correcting its

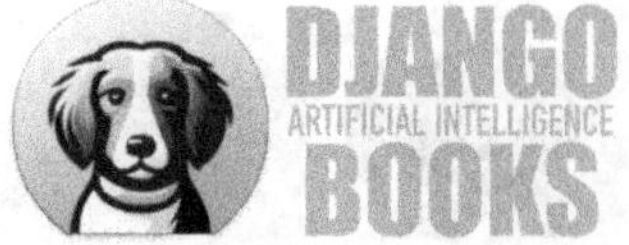

grip or its pace, highlights a unique intergenerational exchange of knowledge and machine learning.

Moreover, the integration of these AI technologies with telehealth services enhances the continuity of care. Physicians and family members can receive updates and alerts, ensuring that any changes in health are promptly addressed. This seamless web of care creates a safety net that comforts not only the elderly but also their families, knowing that their loved ones are under constant, competent care.

In essence, the narrative of care companion robots in elderly care redefines the relationship between technology and aging. It's a story where the cold touch of metal is warmed by the simulated heartbeat of a caring companion, where each algorithmically driven act of assistance is also an act of empathy. As this chapter unfolds, readers are not merely informed about technological advancements but are invited to envision a future where aging is embraced with dignity, independence, and a dose of delightful companionship, all facilitated by the compassionate capabilities of AI.

In the wondrous world where artificial intelligence melds with the mysteries of the human mind, particularly in

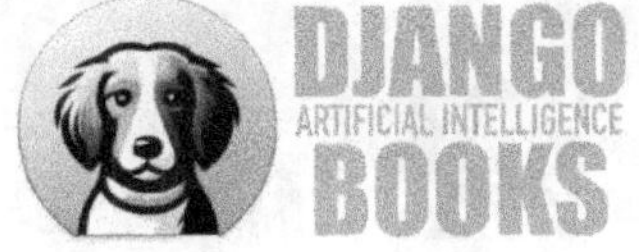

the realm of aging, a remarkable development unfolds in the form of memory maintenance mechanisms. This innovative application of AI not only fortifies the faculties of the mind against the ravages of time but does so with a deftness that imbues the daily lives of the elderly with a renewed sense of vitality and vibrancy. Far from being mere figments of futuristic fiction, these mechanisms are grounded in today's technology, offering practical, tangible benefits that can significantly enhance the cognitive conservation of aging populations.

Delightfully, imagine an AI system that acts as a digital diary, meticulously logging daily experiences and interactions. This isn't just any diary, however; it's equipped with cognitive computing capabilities that can highlight memories based on emotional content or personal significance. The whimsy of this system lies in its ability to prompt the user with forgotten memories, perhaps bringing up the anniversary of a joyous family gathering or a forgotten favorite song, thereby weaving a rich tapestry of past experiences into the present moment. This serves not only to delight but to actively combat the onset of cognitive

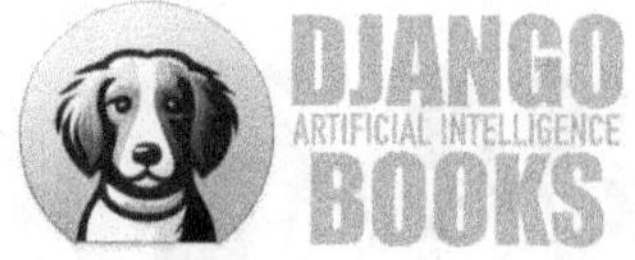

decline by keeping the brain actively engaged with its own history.

Furthermore, AI's role extends into more sophisticated realms, such as the direct stimulation of neurological pathways involved in memory retention and recall. Through non-invasive techniques like transcranial magnetic stimulation, AI-guided devices can help maintain and even enhance neural efficiency in a targeted manner. Picture a scenario where, at scheduled times, a device gently stimulates specific brain regions to enhance synaptic connectivity, all while the user enjoys a morning cup of tea or reads the newspaper. The notion that one's morning routine could subtly include a session of neural upkeep might elicit a chuckle, yet the profound impact of such regular cognitive care is no laughing matter.

Moreover, AI systems integrate seamlessly with therapeutic routines designed to halt or reverse cognitive decline. These systems use predictive analytics to tailor cognitive exercises that are not only based on the user's medical history but also dynamically adjusted according to daily performance metrics on memory-related tasks. The system might suggest puzzles, memory games, or even virtual reality experiences that are both enjoyable and

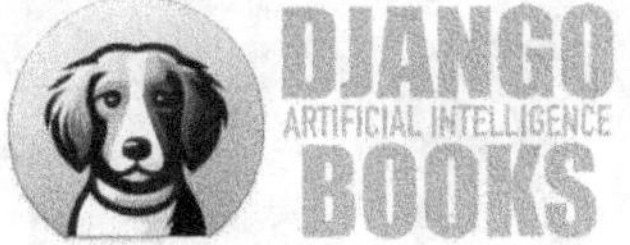

beneficial. Imagine a virtual reality game designed to mimic a historical event, accidentally teaching grandparents more about techno music than the Treaty of Versailles, yet each interaction is carefully crafted to strengthen cognitive pathways.

Additionally, AI-powered memory maintenance also facilitates social interactions, which are crucial for mental health and cognitive longevity. Through social platforms integrated with AI, users can connect with peers sharing similar interests, participate in group activities, or engage in virtual gatherings that stimulate memory and conversation. The amusement in a group of octogenarians animatedly discussing their virtual travels or competing in an AI-curated quiz cannot be overstated.

Lastly, the integration of these AI systems in everyday environments ensures that elderly users can maintain their independence longer, with AI assistants providing gentle reminders for medication, appointments, or staying active. The mix of an AI assistant gently prodding one to water the plants—lest they suffer a fate similar to the forgotten cacti of last summer—blends practicality with making daily routines both manageable and enjoyable.

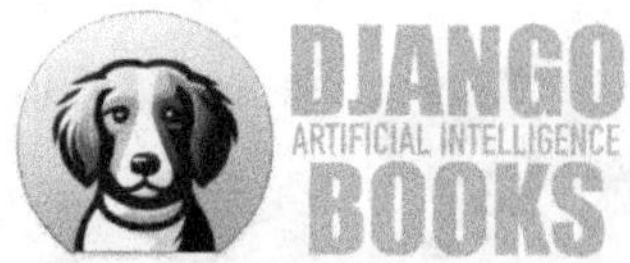

As this chapter elucidates, the intersection of AI and cognitive conservation is not merely about maintaining memory but enriching the lives of those who may feel their memories slipping away. It offers a beacon of hope, harnessing cutting-edge technology to ensure that every golden year is lived with dignity, independence, and a continued joy for life, punctuated by moments of learning, all under the watchful guidance of artificial intelligence.

As we embark on the splendidly sophisticated sojourn into the realm of senescence, where time's inexorable passage etches its evidence upon the human form, artificial intelligence emerges as a beacon of bespoke guardianship. This sentinel of senescence, through an intricate network of sensors and solutions, offers not merely tracking but also targeted interventions for age-related ailments, thus transforming the twilight years into a period marked by sustained vitality and diminished debilitation. The integration of AI into the daily lives of the aging population allows for a proactive approach to health management, where the subtleties of senescence are neither surprises nor inevitabilities but challenges to be met with precise and personalized care.

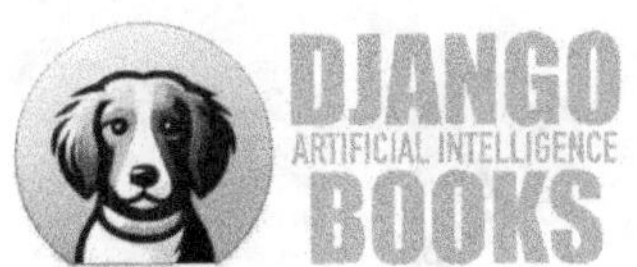

My Health Enhanced by Artificial Intelligence

Envision a scenario rich with the romance of technology and the rigor of real-world application: sensors seamlessly woven into the fabric of daily life, perhaps embedded within the walls of one's home or the very clothing upon one's back. These vigilant sentinels continuously collect data on vital signs, movement patterns, and even subtle changes in routine that might indicate health issues brewing beneath the surface. With the finesse of a fine-tuned orchestra, AI analyzes this deluge of data, discerning patterns and predicting potential problems before they burgeon into crises. The charm in this high-tech tale is palpable, as one imagines an elderly individual playfully scolding their overly attentive smart sweater for fussing about their slightly elevated heart rate during a particularly suspenseful television drama.

Moreover, the potential of AI in this arena extends into the development of customized treatment protocols, tailored to the individual's specific physiological and psychological profile. For example, AI can optimize medication schedules based on the user's activity levels and sleep patterns, ensuring maximum efficacy and minimal side effects. The irony of a machine fine-tuning human function is not lost in this narrative, as it highlights

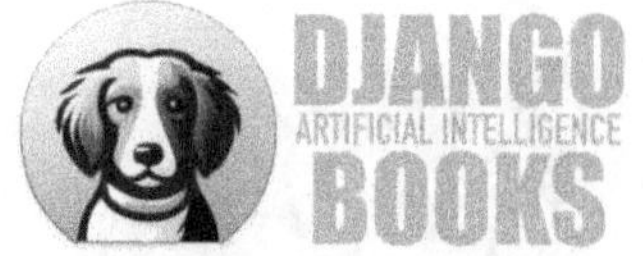

how our own creations come to care for us, with a mix of maternal meticulousness and mechanical efficiency.

Additionally, AI's capability to interact with healthcare providers offers a seamless bridge between personal health monitoring and professional medical intervention. Should an anomaly or ailment be detected, AI systems can alert medical personnel, providing them with detailed data that can inform further diagnostics and treatments. This not only enhances the efficiency of medical care but also embeds a layer of emotional security, knowing that one's health is under constant surveillance by a cybernetic guardian.

Furthermore, these senescence sensors and their accompanying solutions are instrumental in fostering independence among the elderly, reducing the need for constant human supervision while maintaining an optimal level of care. The magic of an elderly person negotiating with their AI for an extra hour past their recommended bedtime or a cheeky indulgence in a forbidden treat captures the blend of control and care that AI brings into their lives.

Thus, as this narrative unfolds, we delve deeper into a future where aging is not a curse to be borne but a process

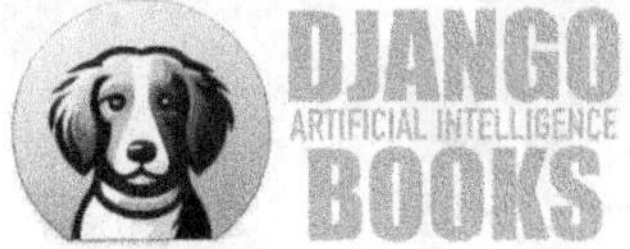

to be managed with grace and acuity. AI, in its role as both shield and scholar, not only protects but also educates us on the possibilities of maintaining health and happiness far into our later years. This topic does not merely inform but inspires, offering a vision of a future where the golden years are both lengthened and enriched, thanks not to the mythical fountains of youth but to the tangible technologies of today. Here, every sensor and solution not only adds years to life but life to years, ensuring that age remains but a number, not a sentence.

As we approach the solemn shores of life's final chapter, the role of artificial intelligence in end-of-life care unfolds as a narrative of dignity, design, and data-driven compassion. In this sensitive stage, AI becomes not merely a tool of technological utility but a profound partner in crafting a close of life that respects the individual's desires and dignity while providing comfort and care. The deployment of AI in this delicate domain reveals a commitment to enhancing life quality even as it wanes, ensuring that the twilight of human existence is both honored and handled with an astuteness that only sophisticated systems can provide.

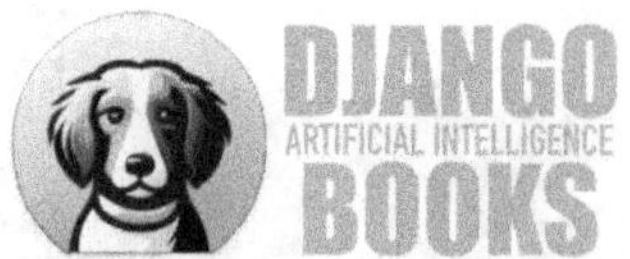

Envision a scenario where AI systems, through their meticulous matrix of sensors and software, monitor the health conditions of terminally ill patients with unobtrusive precision. These systems are capable of detecting even the subtlest changes in patient comfort and symptom severity, enabling timely and tailored interventions. One might wryly remark upon the irony of having spent a lifetime fearing technology's takeover, only to find in its hands a gentle guidance through life's final journey. Here, AI proves itself not as an overlord of our fears but as an oracle of comfort, managing medication schedules, environmental settings, and even interaction timings to suit the patient's preferences and needs.

The design aspect of AI in end-of-life care involves creating interactive environments that respond to the cognitive and emotional states of the patient. For instance, AI-driven systems can modulate room lighting, play soothing music, or display serene landscapes, transforming a sterile hospital room into a place of peace and personalization. The notion of a room that changes its scenery based on whether it's drama or tranquility you need might bring a smile, even in challenging times,

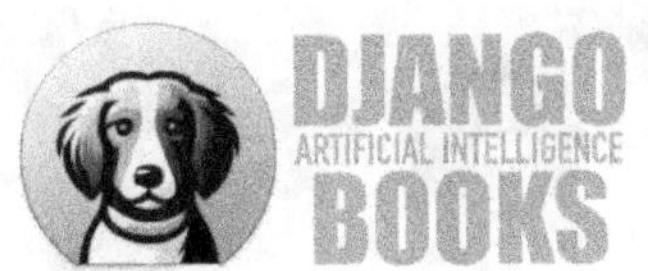

underscoring the nuanced understanding AI holds over human emotions.

Furthermore, AI contributes significantly to maintaining dignity in end-of-life scenarios by enabling patients to communicate their needs and desires more effectively, even as their ability to communicate conventionally wanes. Advanced speech recognition and predictive text algorithms can help patients express their thoughts and wishes, thereby actively participating in their care decisions. The subtlety in having a machine better understand your needs than your own kin is both poignant and pointed, reminding us of the depth of data-driven empathy.

Moreover, AI's analytical prowess offers a vault of valuable insights for healthcare providers, delivering comprehensive reports on patient progress and palliative care effectiveness. This facilitates a more informed approach to symptom management and decision-making, tailored to the unique needs of each patient. It's as if the medical team has been gifted a crystal ball, revealing the hidden nuances of care that make all the difference between a day spent in distress and one spent in dignified tranquility.

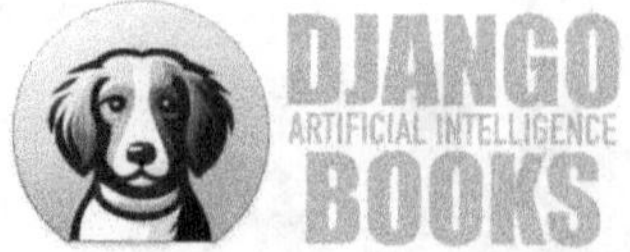

In this sensitive context, AI also supports family members and caregivers by providing them with updates and educational resources, helping them understand the complex processes involved in end-of-life care. The bittersweet aspect here emerges as caregivers find their roles reversed, now guided by the gentle hand of an AI that patiently explains the intricacies of care protocols and medical jargon with the ease of a seasoned teacher.

Thus, as we explore the use of AI in end-of-life care, the narrative weaves a compassionate tale of technology's tender touch in the twilight of life. It is a story that marries the might of machine learning with the mildness of human mercy, ensuring that the journey's end is faced not with fear but with a fortified spirit, supported by sophisticated systems designed to deliver dignity, design, and data-driven care. This chapter is not just a discussion of technological possibilities but a testament to the profound potential of AI to transform the most delicate moments of human existence into periods of peace and personal significance.

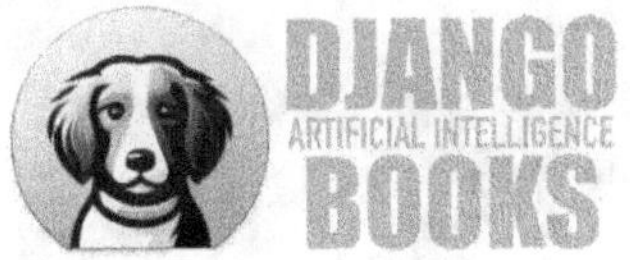

Please Leave a Review

Hey there, savvy reader! If this book is helping you enhance your health with a dash of AI magic, why not take a moment to sprinkle some karma into the universe? Your review could be just what future readers need to discover this gem. It doesn't have to be a novel—just a few seconds for a few words will do!

Simply click the link or point your phone at the QR code. Thanks in advance for sharing your thoughts—trust me, your good health karma is about to skyrocket!!

Click Here to Leave Review

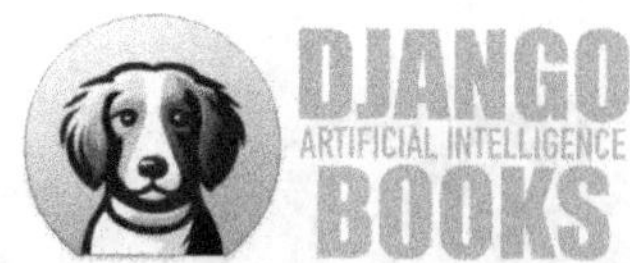

Chapter 8: Navigating AI Healthcare Systems

As we delve into the digital depths of AI healthcare systems, discerning which software sails beyond the sea of sameness becomes essential. For the health-conscious consumer, the quest to select sublime software is not just about purchasing a product; it's about partnering with a platform that promises precision, personalization, and paramount privacy. This topic guides the reader through the labyrinth of available AI health technologies, highlighting the hallmarks of high-quality systems that can truly transform personal health management.

When selecting AI health technology, the first criterion is precision. A system that boasts of sophisticated algorithms must demonstrate an ability to process and analyze health data with pinpoint accuracy. This precision ensures that the recommendations and insights provided are not just generic guidelines but customized strategies tailored to the individual's unique physiological profile. One might find it amusingly paradoxical that in our quest for personal health, our best guides are not human but digital;

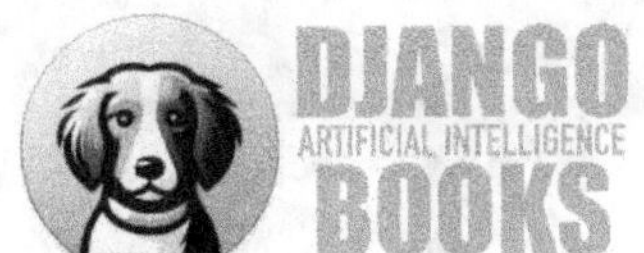

yet, it is this very AI that can discern patterns in data that even the most trained eyes might miss.

The second criterion involves the software's ability to integrate diverse data sources. An exemplary AI health system should harmoniously handle data from electronic health records, wearable device outputs, genetic information, and even environmental factors. The sheer comedy of imagining a system meticulously meshing together your genetic data with the number of steps you took today to suggest a slight adjustment in your dinner's carb content might bring a smile, yet this is the level of detailed dedication that sets superior systems apart.

Adaptability is a key feature of standout AI health technology. The ideal system should not only adapt its recommendations based on new health data but also learn from the outcomes of its advice. For instance, if a dietary adjustment led to improved energy levels or better sleep, the system should incorporate this feedback into future recommendations. The delightful irony of having our technological creations continually learning from us, thereby becoming ever more skilled in managing our health, adds a layer of futuristic fineship to our daily lives.

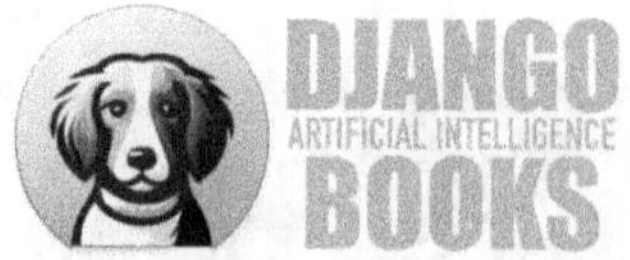

A sublime AI health tech experience is heavily reliant on the user interface. The software must offer a clean, intuitive interface that makes navigation simple for all users, regardless of their tech-savviness. An advanced AI system, capable of complex data analysis, yet unable to provide a user-friendly interface would be akin to having a digital doctor with poor bedside manners; impressive but impractical.

Finally, and perhaps most critically, is the issue of privacy and security. A trustworthy AI health system must ensure that all personal data is protected with the highest standards of security. It should comply with relevant health data protection regulations and be transparent about data usage policies. The notion that your health data could be better traveled than you are—should it ever leak—provides a stark reminder of the need for stringent security measures.

By evaluating AI health technology against these criteria, users can make informed decisions about which systems align best with their personal health goals and ethical standards. This guidance not only serves to educate but also empowers readers, providing them with the tools to harness the benefits of AI in a manner that is safe,

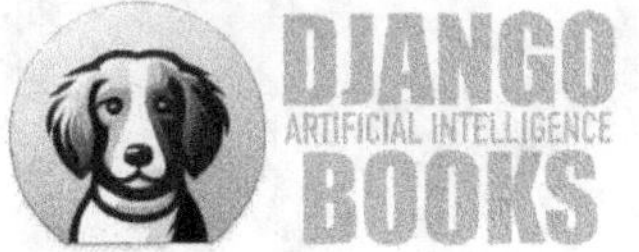

effective, and aligned with their health aspirations. As we explore these systems, we not only advance our understanding of what makes software sublime but also enhance our ability to interact with these digital entities in ways that enrich our health and our lives.

Navigating the nexus of artificial intelligence and personal healthcare practices is akin to embarking on a thrilling odyssey through uncharted technological terrain, where each discovery could significantly amplify one's health and well-being. The integration of AI into personal healthcare practices is not merely a matter of employing sophisticated software but involves embracing a symbiosis of machine learning and daily health habits. This journey enriches the individual's lifestyle, enhances health monitoring precision, and engenders a proactive approach to well-being that is as engaging as it is efficacious.

Embarking on this odyssey requires an initial acclimatization to the idea that one's digital companion could know more about their physiological processes than they do themselves. It's an amusing thought, that a device strapped to your wrist might have a better grasp of your heart rate zones than your own subjective feelings could provide. The first step in this integration process involves

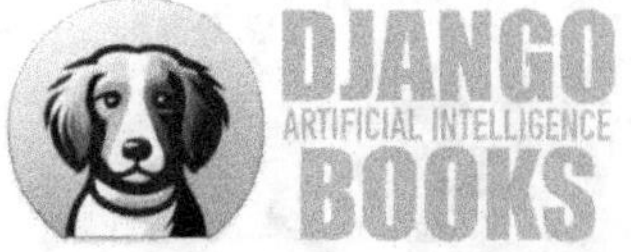

selecting AI tools that align seamlessly with individual health goals, be it managing a chronic condition, optimizing physical fitness, or ensuring mental well-being.

The real magic begins with the customization capabilities of AI. Here, AI shines by providing tailored health monitoring and intervention strategies that adapt over time. For instance, AI-driven applications can analyze data from your fitness tracker, combine it with your dietary inputs, and suggest personalized meal plans and workout routines. The charm of having a virtual nutritionist and personal trainer rolled into one, always ready with a quip about your calorie count or a jest as you jog, transforms mundane health routines into a delightful dialogue with your digital aide.

A pivotal element in this integration is the continuous feedback loop maintained by AI systems. As you interact with these technologies, they learn from your behaviors and refine their advice, creating a cycle of improvement that feels almost like having a conversation with a wise and witty friend who knows your health intimately. Whether reminding you to hydrate more on a hot day or suggesting a stress relief activity based on your recent sleep patterns,

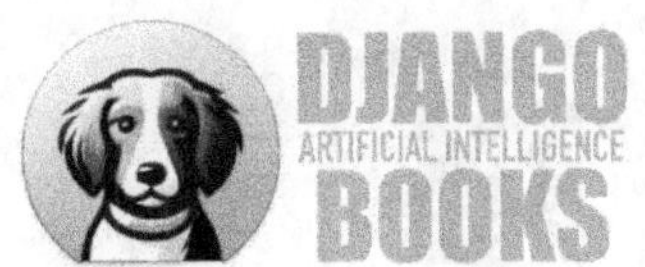

AI becomes a partner in your health journey, to keep the mood light and the advice actionable.

As engaging as these interactions might be, they carry the serious undertone of data security and privacy. Integrating AI into your personal healthcare effectively means ensuring that all your data, from heartbeats to heat maps, is safeguarded with the zeal of a digital fortress. The concept might conjure an image of a digital knight in shining armor, guarding the gates of your personal health data against the marauding invaders of the internet.

Furthermore, AI in personal healthcare acts not only as a monitor and advisor but also as an educator. By providing insights into how different lifestyle choices affect your health, AI systems empower you with knowledge, making health management an enlightening experience. Perhaps, on some idle Tuesday, your AI might casually inform you that the extra cup of coffee is the villain behind your insomnia, presenting this narrative with the gusto of a detective unveiling the culprit in a whodunit.

Thus, as we delve deeper into the topic of integrating AI into personal healthcare practices, we uncover a renaissance in personal health management, where technology meets tenacity, and data delivers daily delights.

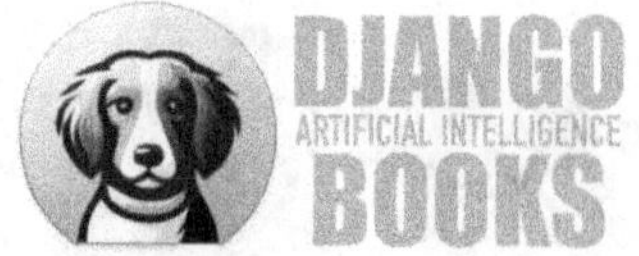

This integration is not just about adopting new tools but about transforming the very fabric of how we view and manage our health. It promises a future where every individual is the master of their own health destiny, guided by the sage advice of their AI companions, who bring wisdom to the wellness journey.

In the increasingly digitized dance of modern healthcare, where algorithms augment and sometimes even automate medical processes, the dynamic between doctor and patient has evolved. Now enters the digital doctor-patient dynamic, a nuanced narrative that demands not only sophistication in technology but also a surplus of trust and transparency. Establishing this trust is pivotal, as the personal data shared is intimate and the stakes, concerning health, are inherently high. This relationship, mediated by machines, must therefore not only be effective but exude a level of earnestness and ethical engagement that engenders confidence and comfort in all involved.

Trust in this context is not merely a matter of faith but is built on the bedrock of transparency and the demonstrable reliability of AI systems. One could whimsically wonder if their digital doc is gossiping about their genetic secrets or pondering personal peccadilloes

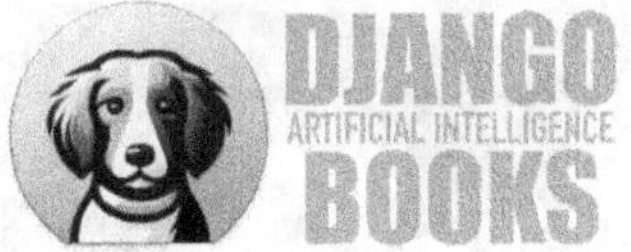

with other programs. However, beyond these playful ponderings lies the serious business of ensuring that AI systems in healthcare are transparent in their operations and decisions. This means that every algorithm must not only perform with precision but also provide patients and doctors with understandable insights into how and why particular medical advice or diagnoses are reached.

Transparency in AI healthcare manifests in several critical areas: the clarity of data usage, the interpretability of algorithmic decisions, and the accountability for the outcomes. For example, when an AI system suggests a particular treatment based on machine learning analysis of patient data, it should be able to show the data and reasoning processes that led to that recommendation. The amusing image of an AI stammering through an explanation in machine language might tickle one's fancy, but in practice, these explanations need to be accessible and comprehensible, not shrouded in computational complexity.

Practically, this means that developers and providers of AI healthcare technologies must prioritize user-friendly interfaces that do not merely spit out decisions or data but do so with clear, actionable explanations. Imagine an AI

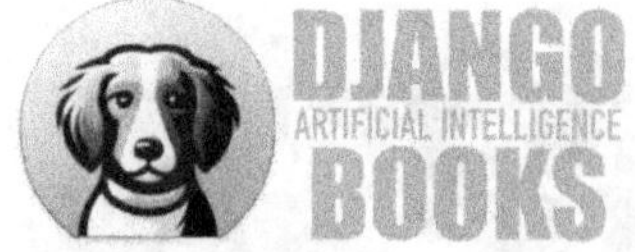

health assistant that not only reminds you to take your medication but explains the impact of missing a dose on your health outcomes in a manner as clear as your pharmacist would, perhaps even with a hint of humor about ensuring you're in top shape for upcoming social shenanigans.

Moreover, this transparency and trust dynamic is crucial for enhancing rather than replacing the traditional doctor-patient relationship. AI should be seen as a bridge, not a barrier, between medical professionals and patients. For instance, when AI is used to diagnose diseases from medical imaging, it can also serve as a tool for doctors to discuss potential treatment paths with patients, using visual aids created by AI to explain complex conditions. The scenario might play out like a tech-savvy medical drama, where the AI highlights areas of concern on scans with the dramatic flair of a detective unveiling clues, making the patient an engaged participant in their healthcare narrative.

To foster trust, healthcare systems must also ensure strict adherence to ethical standards in AI development and deployment, including bias mitigation, privacy protection, and ensuring equity in AI healthcare access. This involves not only technical safeguards but also policy frameworks

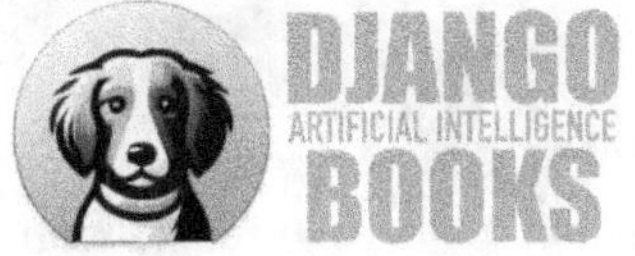

that regulate AI use. The irony of AI potentially serving as both the enforcer and the entity being regulated provides a rich ground for reflection on the future of healthcare governance.

In essence, as we delve into establishing trust through transparency in AI healthcare systems, we are not just exploring a technical requirement but fostering a fundamental human connection. By ensuring that AI systems in healthcare are transparent, we empower patients and professionals alike, making the digital doctor-patient dynamic a duo of delightful, dedicated partners in the dance of modern medicine. The goal here is not only to educate but to ensure that readers are equipped to engage with AI healthcare systems in ways that enhance their health and uphold their rights, turning the digital revolution in healthcare into a trusted ally in their medical journeys.

Embarking upon the exhilarating expedition through the ever-evolving ecosystem of AI in healthcare demands not only a keen curiosity but also a commitment to continuous education and engagement. In this high-speed highway of technological transformation, the pace at which advancements occur can dazzle and daunt even the most dedicated devotees of digital developments. Yet, staying

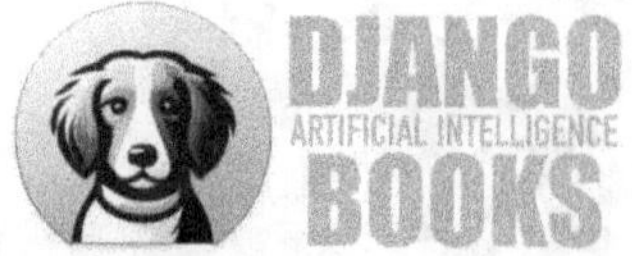

abreast of these changes is crucial, not merely for the sake of knowledge but for actively leveraging these technologies to enhance one's health management practices.

Firstly, understanding the perpetual proliferation of new AI applications within healthcare can seem akin to charting constellations in a rapidly expanding universe. Each new technology, each update, and each breakthrough adds another star to the map, guiding us toward greater health optimization. One could imagine themselves as an intergalactic explorer, toggling through tabs of tech tutorials instead of traversing telescopic territories.

To harness these technologies effectively, one must develop frameworks for fluency in their functionalities. This means not only grasping the basic operating principles but also understanding the implications of their use. For instance, when a new AI-powered diagnostic tool is introduced, one should look beyond the flashy features and delve into the data: How does it improve on previous models? What does it measure, and with what margin of error? Does it integrate seamlessly with existing health monitoring systems? Envisioning oneself in an ongoing

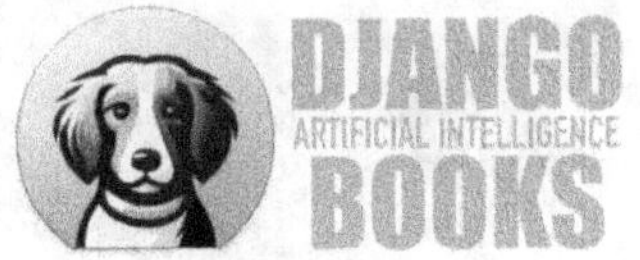

dialogue with developers and devices adds a layer of lively interaction to this educational endeavor.

Engagement with AI technologies is best approached through experiential learning, which could be as simple as participating in virtual webinars, demos, or interactive forums where new AI tools are discussed and demonstrated. One could imagine the occasional clash of cutting-edge computations with commonplace confusions —like accidentally activating voice commands when trying to ask a question during a webinar, only to have both your smartphone and your smart speaker respond simultaneously in a bizarre echo of AI enthusiasm.

Creating a personal learning ecosystem is another vital step. This could involve curating a selection of reliable news sources, subscribing to journals, following thought leaders in AI and healthcare on social media, and even setting up alerts for keywords related to AI advancements that impact your specific health concerns. The whimsy of having your digital devices constantly chirp with cheerful news updates turns the task of keeping up-to-date into a delightful daily discovery.

Furthermore, collaborative learning through community involvement provides a practical and pleasant way to stay

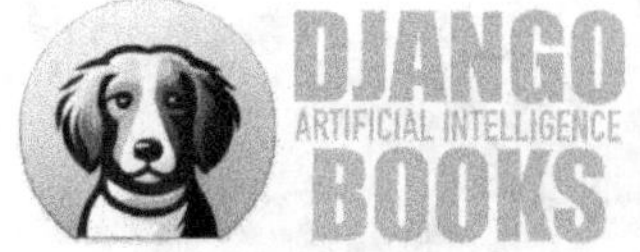

informed. Joining or initiating discussion groups, both online and offline, where individuals share insights and experiences with AI health tech fosters a communal knowledge base that enriches each member. One might find the symphony of syncopated notifications during a heated group chat debate over the best AI fitness trackers, illustrating the lively exchange of ideas and experiences.

Thus, the journey of staying ahead in AI advancements is not a solitary sprint but a collective marathon, punctuated with pit stops of learning and lanes of laughter. It requires a proactive posture, a curious mind, and a joyful engagement with the resources and communities that make navigating this terrain a thrilling adventure. By embracing continuous education and engagement, one not only keeps pace with AI advancements but also enhances their capability to effectively integrate these innovations into their personal health regimen, ensuring that the journey through the landscape of AI healthcare is as enriching as it is exhilarating.

Navigating the intricate legal and insurance landscapes in the context of AI-assisted health is akin to embarking on a formidable quest through a labyrinth of

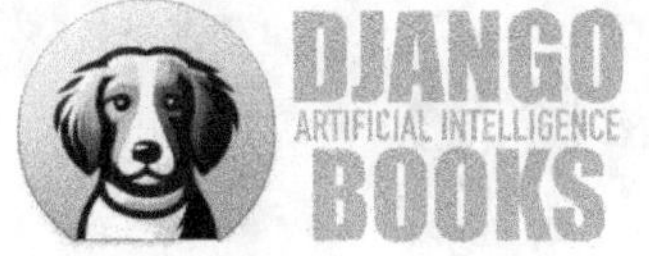

legislative lexicons and insurance intricacies. This journey, crucial for every conscientious consumer of AI healthcare technology, requires a thorough understanding not only of how these technologies impact personal health management but also how they are framed within the broader spectrums of law and insurance. Understanding these frameworks ensures that users can confidently integrate AI into their healthcare regimes, armed with knowledge that protects their rights and maximizes their benefits.

Firstly, delving into the legal dimensions involves untangling the dense thicket of regulations that govern the use of AI in healthcare. Key among these are concerns about data privacy, informed consent, and liability—who is held accountable when AI makes a decision that leads to medical error? The complexity of these questions might bring to mind the byzantine intrigues of medieval courts, where the uninitiated could easily find themselves lost in a maze of legalistic language. It's imperative, therefore, to stay informed about healthcare laws such as HIPAA in the United States, GDPR in Europe, and other similar regulations globally that dictate how personal health information can be collected, used, and shared.

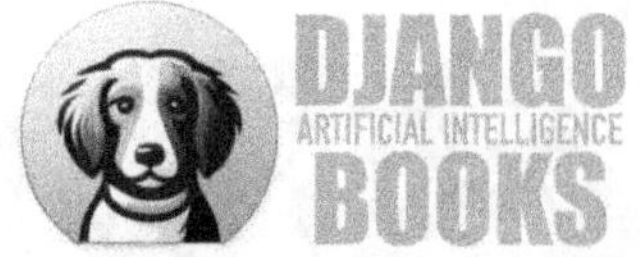

Moving to the insurance implications, one must consider how AI interventions are covered under existing health insurance policies. Are AI-driven diagnostics and treatments considered standard care, and thus reimbursable, or are they regarded as experimental, attracting out-of-pocket expenses? This area often feels like negotiating a bazaar where the value of goods (in this case, AI healthcare services) can vary wildly depending on the insurer's policies. Engaging with insurance providers to understand these nuances can often feel like haggling in an exotic marketplace, albeit less colorful but equally crucial.

Moreover, the rights of patients using AI-enabled health services need clear articulation and staunch advocacy. This involves ensuring that AI systems are not only accurate and safe but also equitable and non-discriminatory in their function. The whimsy of imagining an AI system being put on trial for medical malpractice underscores the serious consideration of how traditional legal concepts like duty of care apply in a world where decisions can be made by algorithms.

To effectively navigate this maze, individuals must become savvy about the specific legal and insurance

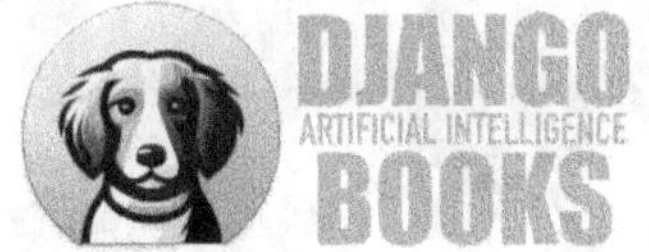

questions relevant to AI in healthcare. This might involve consulting legal experts in healthcare law, engaging with patient advocacy groups, or participating in informational sessions hosted by insurance companies. Envision the proactive health tech user armed with an arsenal of questions, much like a knight with a shield, parrying the blows of potential legal and insurance pitfalls.

Finally, for those particularly invested in the intersection of AI and healthcare, engagement with policymakers and stakeholders offers an avenue to influence how laws and insurance policies evolve in response to new technologies. This participation ensures that the legal and insurance frameworks adapt to better serve the needs of patients while supporting innovation in healthcare. The dynamic of these interactions often resembles a lively debate club, where each participant brings a perspective sharpened by personal experience and professional expertise.

In conclusion, as we explore the legal and insurance landscapes in AI-assisted health, we not only educate ourselves about the current state of affairs but also prepare to actively shape the evolving dialogue around these technologies. This topic not only provides practical insights

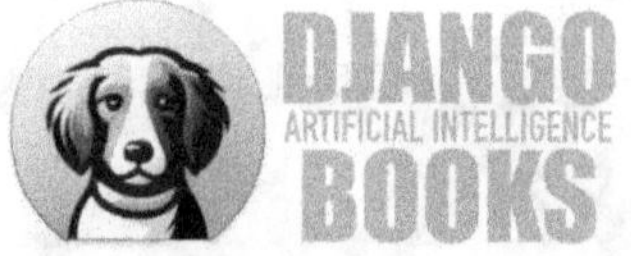

for the reader but also empowers them to navigate these complex terrains with confidence and curiosity, ensuring that their journey through AI healthcare is as secure as it is revolutionary.

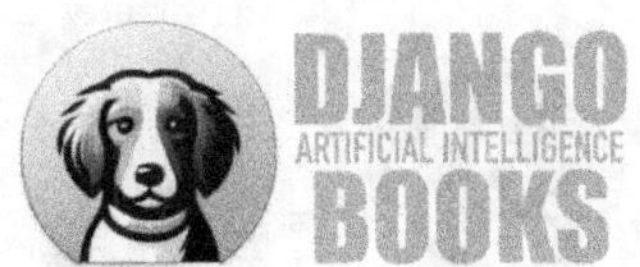

Chapter 9: The Global Impact of AI on Health. Equity, Access, and Ethics

As the tendrils of technology extend across the global health landscape, artificial intelligence stands poised to bridge significant bioinformatics breaches, reducing health disparities that have long marred the medical field. This transformative potential of AI can be leveraged to democratize access to quality healthcare, irrespective of geographical boundaries or socioeconomic statuses. Herein lies a profound exploration of how AI can function not merely as a tool of technological progress but as a beacon of equity, bringing high-level medical expertise to underserved populations and creating a more level playing field in health outcomes across the globe.

AI's capacity to analyze vast datasets can identify health trends and disparities with unprecedented precision. For populations in remote or underserved regions, AI can predict outbreak patterns, optimize resource allocation, and

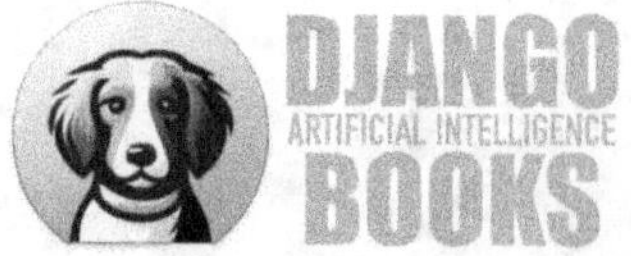

tailor public health interventions based on derived data insights. This approach is akin to having a virtual health overseer who ensures that no area is medically underserved. The integration of AI into these settings often brings a certain humor to the high-tech meets low-tech scenarios, imagining a world-class AI system operating in a rural clinic, where the local healthcare workers are both bemused by and appreciative of its advice.

AI's diagnostic algorithms can process and interpret medical imaging and diagnostic tests faster and often with greater accuracy than human counterparts. By deploying these AI systems in regions with a dearth of trained radiologists or pathologists, patients can receive quicker, more reliable diagnoses. This can be particularly transformative for diseases like tuberculosis or skin cancer, which are prevalent in low-resource settings. The scenario of an AI system spotting diseases from medical images with more flair than a seasoned doctor might seem like a scene from a futuristic film, yet it is rapidly becoming a reality with tangible benefits.

Furthermore, AI can serve as a training and support tool for healthcare providers in underserved areas, augmenting their knowledge and compensating for the lack

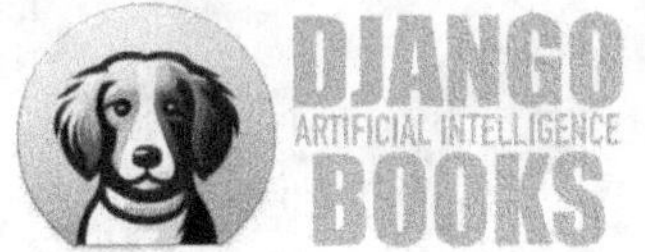

of specialists. Through AI-powered mobile apps or online platforms, local healthcare workers can access up-to-date medical information and training modules, enhancing their ability to provide effective care. The image of a rural healthcare worker consulting an AI on a smartphone about a complex case injects a dose of digital-age reality into traditional medicine, adding both a layer of efficiency and a touch of comedic incongruity.

However, the deployment of AI in such critical roles must be handled with utmost ethical considerations. Issues of privacy, data security, and the potential for AI to unintentionally perpetuate existing biases must be rigorously addressed. This involves designing AI systems that are not only technologically proficient but also culturally sensitive and inclusive. The magic might arise in the form of AI learning local dialects or cultural nuances, navigating language barriers while providing life-saving medical advice.

To maximize the impact of AI on global health equity, collaborations across countries and sectors are essential. These partnerships ensure that innovations are shared and that AI solutions are adapted to fit diverse health ecosystems. The vision of global health leaders and local

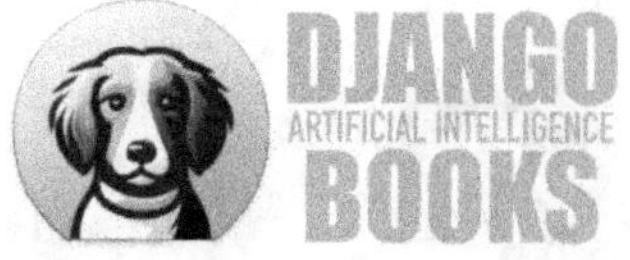

healers coming together, guided by AI, to forge a frontier of fairness in healthcare presents a powerful picture of what is possible when humanity harmonizes with high technology.

As we delve into the potential of AI to bridge the bioinformatics breach and reduce health disparities, we do not merely explore a technological trend but engage with a transformative force capable of reshaping global health landscapes. This discussion offers practical strategies for harnessing AI to ensure that advancements in healthcare reach all corners of the world, transforming the global health dialogue into a narrative of inclusivity, innovation, and integrity.

In the burgeoning field of health AI, the establishment of robust global governance structures is paramount, not only to harness the full potential of these technologies but also to mitigate the risks associated with their widespread implementation. This crucial aspect involves a confluence of policy, privacy, and practice that transcends national boundaries, demanding a cooperative and comprehensive international approach. As we delve into the intricacies of global governance in health AI, it is essential to provide practical ideas that ensure these systems are used ethically, equitably, and effectively, benefiting all of

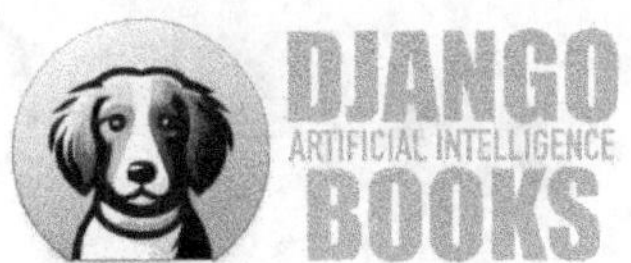

humanity without compromising individual rights and freedoms.

The cornerstone of effective global governance for health AI lies in the development of comprehensive, universally applicable policies. These policies must address a myriad of considerations from ethical usage and data protection to cross-border data flow and interoperability among disparate health systems. For instance, crafting legislation that accommodates both the advanced AI capabilities of developed nations and the burgeoning needs of developing regions requires a nuanced understanding of technology, healthcare, and international law. The complexity of this task is akin to orchestrating a symphony where each nation's laws are an instrument; the challenge lies in creating harmony, not discord.

Privacy protection is particularly paramount in the realm of health AI, where sensitive medical data is an integral part of the technologies' effectiveness. Global governance must therefore establish strict guidelines for data privacy that prevent misuse while enabling the beneficial use of data across international lines. This involves not only technical solutions, such as advanced

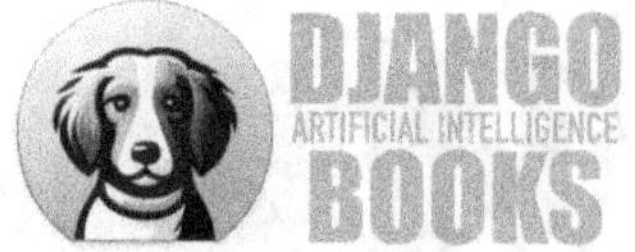

encryption and anonymization techniques but also legal agreements that respect and reflect the diverse privacy cultures of different countries. Imagine navigating a maze where every turn represents a jurisdictional challenge, and every straight path offers a potential for data breach; the goal is to navigate this maze without getting lost or letting the data fall into the wrong hands.

Promoting best practices in the deployment and operation of health AI systems globally is crucial. This includes establishing standards for transparency in AI decision-making processes, ensuring systems are understandable and their operations are explainable to users and regulators alike. Additionally, these practices should encourage the development of AI systems that are inherently unbiased and equitable. The notion of AI as a global digital diplomat, negotiating the nuances of national healthcare policies and practices, offers a light-hearted view of a deeply serious subject.

Effective governance of health AI requires unprecedented levels of international collaboration. This includes sharing research, technologies, and strategies to combat global health challenges. International forums and coalitions can play pivotal roles here, facilitating dialogue

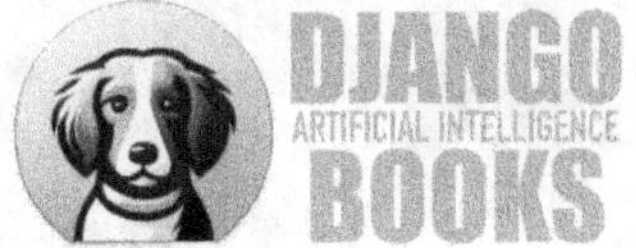

and driving consensus on pressing issues such as intellectual property rights, technology transfer, and capacity building in low-resource settings. The image of AI as a universal language spoken across the globe unites these efforts, symbolizing a collective human endeavor to achieve better health outcomes for everyone, everywhere.

For individuals, understanding and engaging with the global governance of health AI can seem daunting. However, staying informed about international regulations that affect personal data and the AI systems one interacts with is essential. Individuals can also advocate for policies that protect privacy and ensure equity by participating in public consultations and supporting organizations that monitor and influence these areas. By turning the complexities of AI governance into an opportunity for active participation, every person has a chance to shape the landscape of health AI, ensuring it evolves in a manner that is secure, just, and beneficial.

In conclusion, navigating the global governance of health AI involves more than understanding technological capabilities; it requires a concerted effort to build frameworks that uphold ethical standards, protect individual rights, and foster international cooperation. This chapter

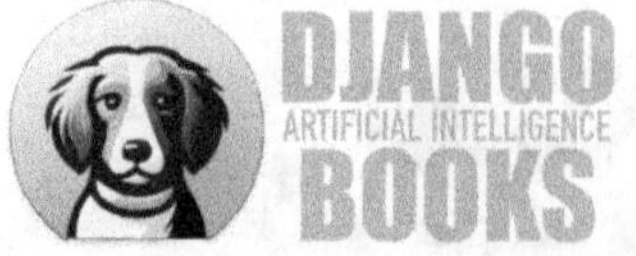

not only provides an in-depth look at the challenges and opportunities of global governance but also offers practical advice on how individuals can contribute to and benefit from these efforts, making the global impact of AI on health a shared and equitable reality.

In the grand tapestry of global healthcare, where disparities loom as large as the diseases they accompany, artificial intelligence has emerged as a knight in digital armor, equipped with altruistic algorithms designed to extend the reach of humanitarian healthcare. These algorithms are not merely lines of code but lifelines cast across the digital divide, reaching out to underserved populations with a precision and perspicacity previously unattainable. This exploration dives deep into how AI's philanthropic prowess is not only leveling the playing field but also changing the game entirely in favor of global health equity.

Picture this: remote villages where healthcare workers are as rare as a rainy day in the desert, now having the power of AI at their fingertips. These AI systems can analyze symptoms, suggest treatments, and predict outbreaks before they burgeon into full-blown epidemics. The humor in the situation might stem from a villager's

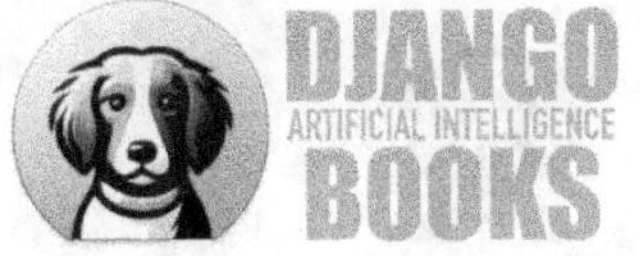

baffled reaction to a tablet dictating treatment protocols in the local dialect, surprised that a device so small could be so wise. Yet, behind the chuckles lies a profound transformation in healthcare delivery, making quality medical advice accessible at the tap of a screen.

The democratization of diagnostics through AI, particularly in areas plagued by poverty and inaccessible healthcare, is akin to distributing magic glasses that can see into the body, revealing the hidden ailments within. These AI-driven diagnostic tools can interpret X-rays, MRIs, and other medical images with astonishing accuracy, often surpassing the local medical expertise available. The irony of an algorithm in Silicon Valley diagnosing a farmer in Sub-Saharan Africa is not lost on us; it's a peculiar twist of fate where technology transcends geography to touch lives.

Furthermore, AI's role in predicting and managing epidemic outbreaks is a narrative straight out of a science fiction novel turned reality. Using data from various sources, including satellite imagery, mobile health data, and real-time disease reporting, AI models can predict the spread of diseases like malaria or dengue fever with eerie accuracy. It's as if the AI has a crystal ball, forecasting the

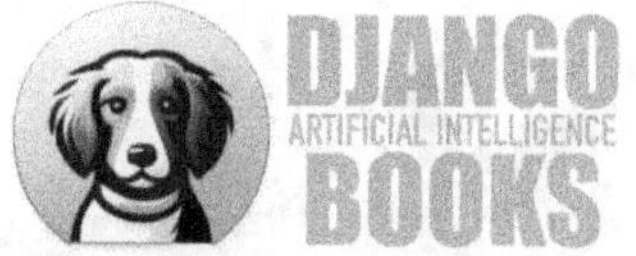

future of public health, and decides to write a thriller where it's the hero that saves the day before the villain even knows the plot.

Resource allocation, especially in crisis scenarios, can often feel like a high-stakes poker game, where every decision impacts lives. Here, AI steps in as the ace up the sleeve, analyzing needs and optimizing the distribution of medical supplies, vaccines, and personnel. The quirkiness of AI playing logistician might conjure images of robots racing down hospital halls, distributing supplies with robotic efficiency, but the reality is a system that ensures no resource is wasted, and no patient is overlooked.

AI's deployment in such varied and culturally rich settings also brings to the forefront the need for culturally sensitive and ethical programming. The algorithms must not only be altruistic but also attuned to the cultural nuances and ethical considerations of the regions they serve. The amusing paradox of teaching a machine about human culture underscores the complexity of AI's role in humanitarian healthcare—it must be as wise as a sage and as humble as a student, continually learning from and adapting to the global stage it acts upon.

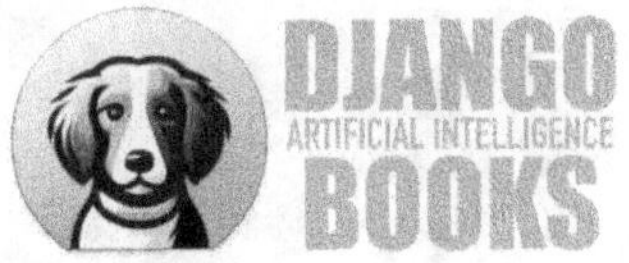

In sum, as we unpack the narrative of AI's altruistic algorithms and their role in humanitarian healthcare, we are not just reviewing technological advancements; we are witnessing a revolution in how care is conceived and delivered globally. This exploration is laden with practical insights for engaging with and advancing this technology, ensuring that as AI reshapes healthcare, it does so with a heart as well as a mind, proving that the most sophisticated algorithms can also be the most compassionate.

The ethical exportation of AI technology in the realm of global health care is akin to navigating a high-seas adventure where the winds of innovation must be balanced against the buoys of bioethics. As nations and corporations hoist the sails of AI solutions across international waters, the compass of morality must guide them to ensure that these technological treasures do not become the modern-day equivalents of colonial conquests but are instead beacons of beneficence.

Embarking on this venture requires a keen understanding that while AI technology holds the promise of transforming healthcare landscapes globally, its deployment must be approached with both cultural sensitivity and regulatory savvy. Picture this: a world where

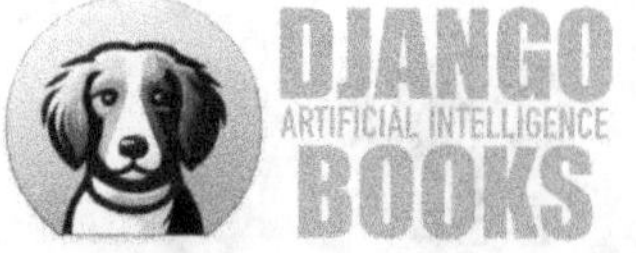

AI health technologies are as commonly exchanged as spices once were along the Silk Road. However, instead of merely trading goods, we're exchanging life-altering capabilities and ethical considerations. Imagine an AI system designed in Silicon Valley trying to navigate the bustling streets of Bangkok, offering dietary advice that humorously misinterprets local cuisine preferences.

The creation of cross-continental guidelines for the deployment of AI in healthcare involves not just an alignment of technical standards but also an ethical alignment. It is essential to ensure that AI applications respect the local customs, traditions, and needs of their new homes. The quirkiness of an AI system learning to adapt to local dialects and health belief models adds a layer of charm to the clinical precision of healthcare, offering moments of levity and learning as the AI adjusts its protocols from sushi to schnitzel, or from preventative measures for tropical diseases to those more common in temperate climes.

As these AI systems cross borders, the balance between their benefits and the boundaries of ethical use becomes crucial. There must be robust frameworks in place to prevent the exploitation of data and to ensure that

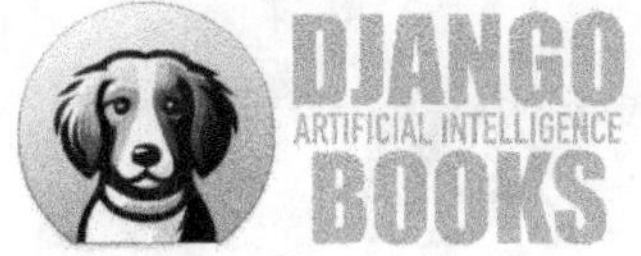

the benefits of AI technologies are equitably distributed. Imagine an AI designed to diagnose skin conditions being introduced to regions with vastly different demographic profiles than those it was trained on; the humor—and challenge—lies in teaching the AI the nuances of dermatological diversity.

Transparency in how AI technologies are developed, trained, and deployed plays a critical role in building trust. This involves not just open communication about the capabilities and limitations of AI systems but also about who stands to benefit from their use. There is an amusing irony in the idea of an AI system having to openly admit its shortcomings in understanding local medical practices, much like a foreign medical student on their first day of rounds in a new country.

Finally, empowering local stakeholders by involving them in the development and customization of AI applications ensures that the exportation of such technology is beneficial and not merely extractive. This is where the real magic happens: local healthcare providers collaborate with AI developers to create tailored solutions that respect local nuances and maximize local benefits. The spectacle of local health workers educating a

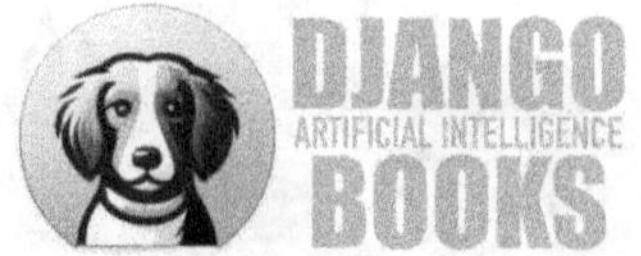

sophisticated AI system in the ways of indigenous medicine could provide both relief and critical insight into the successful integration of AI into diverse healthcare systems.

In conclusion, as we weave through the topic of ethical exportation of AI technology, we transform from mere observers into active participants in a narrative that is as rich and complex as it is critical. This chapter not only informs but inspires readers to consider how AI can be both a universal helper and a culturally competent caretaker, ensuring that as AI solutions travel, they carry with them the standards of equity, ethics, and respect that are the hallmarks of truly transformative technology.

Navigating the nuanced narrative of artificial intelligence in global healthcare invites an exploration into the dual domains of universal utility and localized logic. This intricate dance between broad applicability and cultural specificity underscores the necessity for AI systems to be not only globally competent but also intimately acquainted with local customs, languages, and medical practices. As we delve into this dynamic, we unveil the complexities and comedic contrasts that arise when high-tech healthcare meets diverse cultural landscapes.

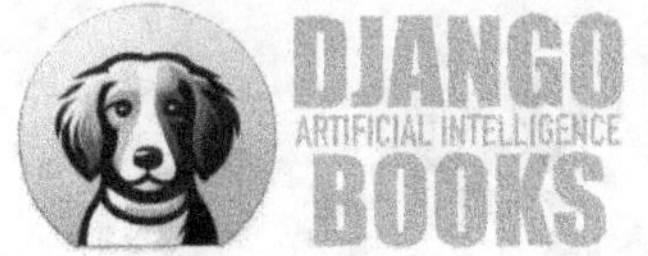

The endeavor to imbue AI with universal utility—making it a tool as versatile as a Swiss Army knife but as precise as a scalpel—presents a unique set of challenges and opportunities. The idea of an AI system trained on vast global data sets offers the tantalizing promise of a tool that can diagnose diseases from Detroit to Dhaka with equal adeptness. However, the a buffled eyebrow may be rised when this globally minded AI encounters local dialects, mistaking a benign colloquialism for a clinical symptom, leading to diagnoses that are as hilariously off mark as a novice trying to perform a tango after a single dance lesson.

On the flip side, instilling localized logic within AI systems necessitates a deep dive into the cultural context in which healthcare is delivered. This means programming AI not only with languages but with an understanding of regional medical ethics, traditional remedies, and patient treatment preferences. Imagine an AI carefully suggesting traditional herbal remedies in an area renowned for its high-tech pharmaceutical industry, or vice versa, recommending advanced biotech solutions to a community where herbal teas are the go-to cure.

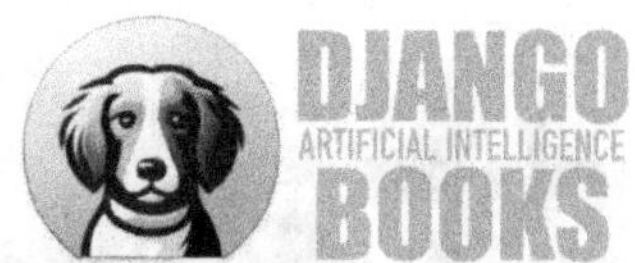

The balancing act involves a sophisticated synthesis of integrating universal medical standards with local healthcare needs. For instance, an AI system might be adept at spotting patterns indicative of a certain disease that it learned from a global dataset but must adapt its recommendations to align with local medical resources and patient preferences. It's akin to an AI chef who can cook any cuisine in the world but needs to know whether the locals prefer spicy or mild, sweet or savory, not to end up serving hot chili sauce to someone expecting a mild tomato dip.

Training AI for cultural competence involves an iterative process of learning and adjustment. This includes feeding it with region-specific data and outcomes to refine its algorithms—a task that might remind one of training a parrot to speak different languages, only to find it humorously mixes them up at a diplomatic dinner.

Furthermore, the ethical implications and policy considerations in deploying culturally competent AI in healthcare cannot be overstated. Ensuring that AI respects patient privacy, consent, and delivers care that is ethically aligned with local customs requires ongoing oversight and regulation. The whimsy of international AI health

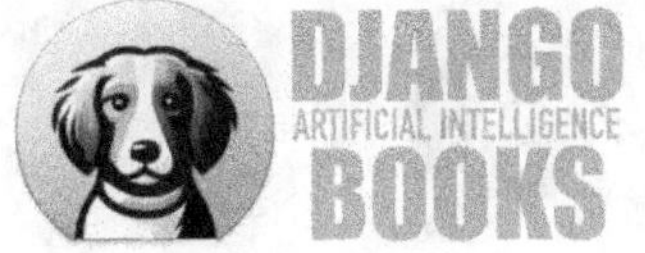

regulations could be compared to an elaborate dance of diplomats, each trying to sync their steps without stepping on each other's toes.

As this exploration of the cultural competence of AI in healthcare unfolds, it reveals that the path to harmonizing universal utility with localized logic is fraught with challenges but also filled with immense potential. This journey does not merely adjust the settings on a global machine but reprograms it to resonate with the rhythms of local life. By embracing both the universal capabilities and the unique cultural contexts of AI application in healthcare, we pave the way for a future where artificial intelligence can serve humanity with both widespread wisdom and local love, ensuring that every laugh shared in the understanding of its use is as heartfelt as the care it provides.

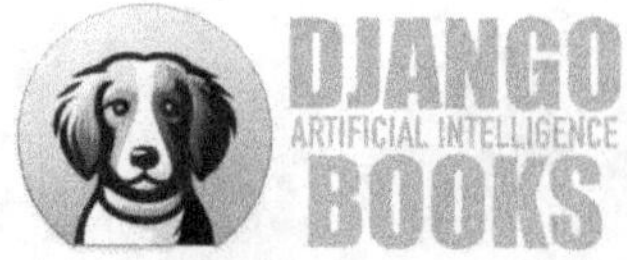

Chapter 10: The Future Foretold, Next-Generation Innovations in AI Health

Ah, diving into the abyss of health-enhancing prospects facilitated by nascent artificial intelligence technologies provides a panorama of untold possibilities where one can scarcely distinguish between the wild conjectures of a sci-fi aficionado and the earnest prognostications of the venerated science savants. As we pirouette through this caleidoscopic futurescape of health innovations, let us delicately unravel the speculative yet tantalizing threads of future AI systems that promise to catapult our mundane existence into a veritable utopia of wellness and longevity.

Imagine, if you will, an AI so seamlessly integrated into your daily regimen that it not only monitors every heartbeat with the precision of a Swiss watchmaker but also anticipates potential maladies with the prophetic acuity of an oracle. This isn't merely about wearing a fitness tracker

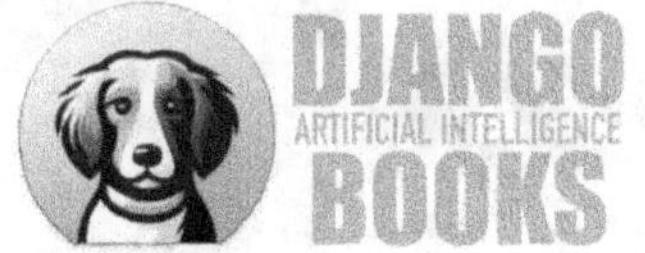

that nudges you to climb ten more stairs; this is about a symbiotic AI companion that knows you more intimately than you know yourself. It configures your diet based on your genomic data, your past meal preferences, and the subtle nuances of your body's real-time nutritional demands, all while making the food appear as palatable as if a Michelin-star chef had a hand in its creation.

Envision further, an AI dermatologist, nonpareil, a virtuoso of virtual skin care, perpetually at your beck and call. This digital dermatologist doesn't merely analyze your skin type or recommend sunscreen; it synthesizes data from a panoply of sources—your genetic predispositions, the precise pollutant levels in your immediate environment, even your stress levels gleaned from your latest social media tirades—and concocts a personalized skin regimen that ensures your visage remains as effulgent as a youth in the bloom of health.

Then, there's the AI mental health guru, an entity not confined by the traditional paradigms of psychiatry or the static words of printed self-help tomes. This AI, equipped with algorithms that probably have more empathy than the average human, could provide real-time mental health assistance. Imagine an AI that crafts bespoke therapeutic

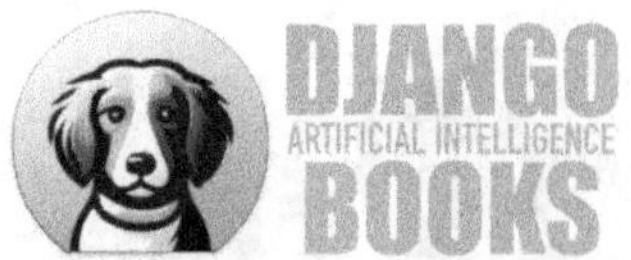

sessions based on your current mental state, drawing from a vast expanse of psychological strategies and therapeutic practices, ensuring each session is as refreshing as a sojourn to a serene oasis in a desolate desert.

Not to be outdone by its digital compatriots, envision an AI pharmaceutical savant, a maestro of molecular concoctions, capable of designing personalized medications. This AI doesn't merely suggest generic prescriptions but synthesizes drugs tailored to the unique biochemical landscape of your body. Each pill or potion is not only concocted to combat your current ailment but also optimized to synergize with everything from your gut bacteria to your last ingested meal, ensuring efficacy and minimizing side effects.

Last, imagine a future where AI transcends its role as a mere facilitator of health and becomes an architect of human enhancement. Here, AI systems could potentially orchestrate the very building blocks of life to craft versions of us that are not only free from diseases but also endowed with capabilities that extend the very definitions of human potential. This could range from enhanced cognitive abilities allowing for profound intellectual endeavors to

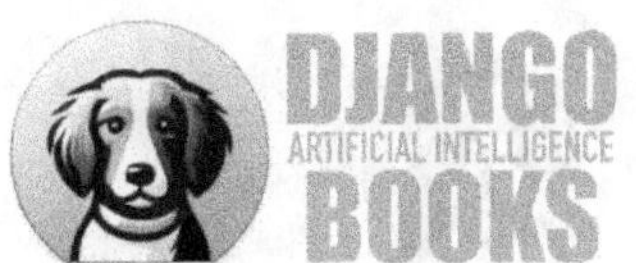

physical enhancements enabling feats that today exist only in the realm of superheroes.

As we teeter on the brink of these groundbreaking innovations, it's critical to anchor our exhilaration in the bedrock of ethical consideration and practical utility. The future depicted here is speculative, yes, but it also holds a mirror to the limitless potential of human ingenuity when coupled with the computational might of artificial intelligence. As we march toward this brave new world, let us wield these tools not just with the giddy excitement of a child with a new toy but with the sagacious foresight of stewards destined to forge a healthier, more vibrant future for all.

As we meander further into the labyrinthine possibilities of artificial intelligence and its intermingling with our daily lives, let us consider the prospects of creating hyper-personalized health habitats—an enviable amalgamation of AI and environmental wellness that promises to transmute our living spaces into bastions of health and longevity. The notion of our surroundings being tuned to our health needs might sound like a page torn from a utopian novel, yet the tendrils of current technology hint at such future realities with tantalizing clarity.

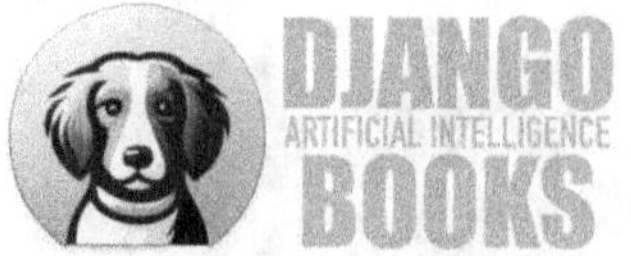

One must first comprehend the monumental potential residing in AI's capability to analyze and respond to environmental factors affecting health. Envision an intelligent habitat that adjusts its parameters not by the whims of a clunky thermostat or the static settings of a humidifier but through the discerning eye of AI that understands your body's current state and its needs to the minutiae. This habitat would control air quality, temperature, lighting, and even acoustic ambiance to optimize your physical and psychological well-being.

Consider the air you breathe, often a cocktail of unseen pollutants and allergens. Here, AI steps in as a vigilant overseer, continuously monitoring air quality and dynamically adjusting air filters and purifiers to eradicate pollutants at the molecular level. Beyond mere purification, imagine this system dispersing nano-scale health enhancers—perhaps vitamins or mood-improving pheromones—transforming every breath into a sigh of relief, literally and metaphorically.

Lighting, too, plays a crucial role in our health, affecting everything from our sleep cycles to our mood. An AI-driven system could orchestrate the lighting in your home not just for aesthetic appeal but as a maestro

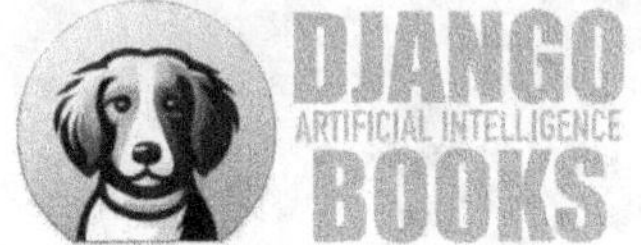

manipulates the orchestra for peak performance—altering wavelengths and intensity throughout the day to bolster your circadian rhythm, enhance your mood, or increase your productivity. As the sun sets, your personal AI dims the blues and heightens the reds, coaxing your body into a restful readiness for sleep.

Temperature and humidity control also ascend to unprecedented levels of personalization. No longer will homes be slaves to a single central thermostat setting; instead, they will feature zones that adapt in real-time to your body's thermal signature and activity level, enveloping you in a cocoon of comfort that follows you without prompt.

But why stop at mere reactive measures? AI in your health habitat could predictively adjust environments based on both your immediate health data and predictive models of your future state. If the AI anticipates a stressful day ahead, it could increase oxygen levels to boost cognition and alertness, or infuse calming scents if a restful evening is paramount.

Moreover, this environmental symphony is conducted on the grand stage of your overall health data ecosystem. This AI isn't just a standalone maestro but part of an

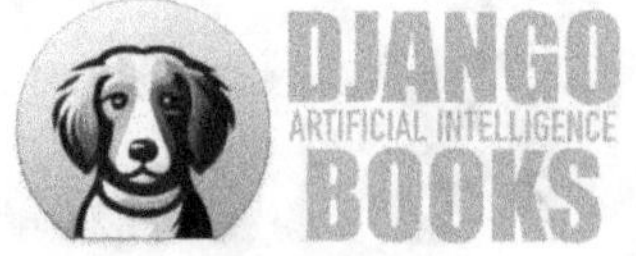

ensemble, communicating with your wearable health monitors, your digital diet assistant, even your AI-enhanced fitness coach, to form a cohesive strategy tailored just for you.

The convergence of AI with our living environments opens a portal to previously uncharted territories of health optimization. These are not merely habitats; they are sanctuaries crafted with the sole intent of fostering an optimal life. As these technologies evolve, so too will our understanding of what it means to live well. Let us stride confidently toward this horizon, with AI as our compass, guiding us to healthier, happier lives in spaces that do more than shelter—they nurture.

Embarking upon the resplendent shores of the quantum realm, where the baffling and mind-bending rules of quantum physics reside, we find a landscape so fertile for hyperbole that even the most flamboyant science fiction writers might blush. Yet, it is in this very realm that quantum computing promises to transform the stalwart domain of healthcare from a merely efficient industry into a veritable wizard of well-being, performing feats that could make even a seasoned magician drop their wand in astonishment.

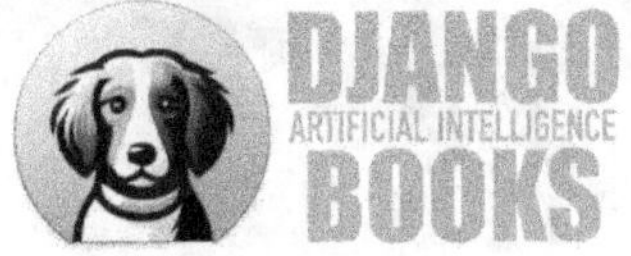

Quantum computing, that bewitching brainchild of quantum mechanics, stands poised to revolutionize healthcare by wielding the double-edged sword of superposition and entanglement. This isn't just a minor upgrade—a mere bump from version 2.0 to 3.0—this is akin to leaping from sending smoke signals to instant messaging across the cosmos. The computational power of quantum computers could decipher the most convoluted biological conundrums.

Imagine, if your cerebrum can handle the gymnastics, a quantum-enhanced AI tasked with mapping the enigmatic labyrinth of human genetics. Traditional computers plod through genetic data like a sloth through molasses, but a quantum computer zips through these calculations with the alacrity of a hare on a caffeine spree. What might take years in computational time could be condensed to mere minutes. The result? Tailored medical treatments that make bespoke Savile Row suits look off-the-rack. You could receive personalized medicine so specific that it knows you better than you know yourself—right down to your last quirky nucleotide.

And what about drug discovery, that arduous, eye-wateringly expensive process that moves slower than a

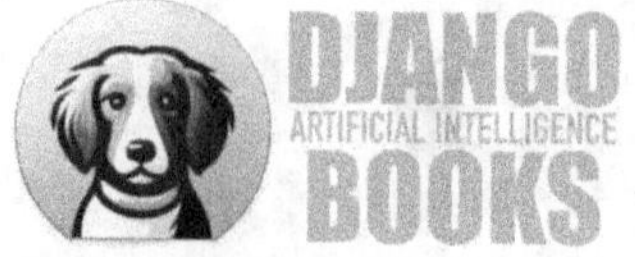

snail on a leisurely stroll? Here, quantum computing dashes in like a superhero, cape billowing, to save the day. By simulating molecular interactions at an unprecedented scale and speed, quantum AI could unearth new therapeutic compounds with the enthusiasm of a child uncovering prizes in a treasure hunt. The pharmacopeia of the future might be so replete with efficacious drugs that even the common cold doesn't stand a chance.

But let's not confine our imaginations to mere processing speed and drug discotheques. The integration of quantum computing into everyday healthcare could usher in diagnostic tools that not only detect diseases at their inception but predict them before they even dare manifest. It's as if your doctor could gaze into a crystal ball, except the crystal ball is a quantum computer, and the mystical fog within is the probabilistic calculations of your future health.

Preventive medicine could reach such dizzying heights of accuracy that your AI-powered health monitors might gently nudge you to adjust your diet or exercise regime decades before any symptoms dare rear their ugly heads. "Eat more kale," it might suggest one morning, "and

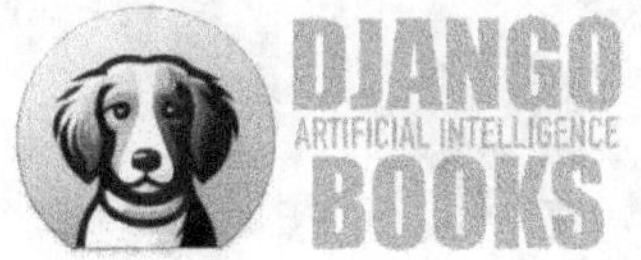

perhaps throw in a jog or two; your heart will thank you in 2045."

In this scintillating vision of the future, as quantum computing and AI converge to elevate healthcare into realms previously relegated to the annals of fantasy, we stand on the cusp of a medical revolution. A revolution not merely of technology but of expectation, where the question shifts from "What can be cured?" to "What can be prevented?" With quantum computing in our arsenal, the future is not just bright; it's dazzling enough to warrant sunglasses. As we chart this audacious course, let's don our proverbial lab coats and top hats, for the magic show—starring quantum computing and healthcare—is about to begin, and it promises to be a spectacle of epic proportions.

As we delve into the arcane yet burgeoning domain where artificial intelligence conjoins with the minuscule marvels of nanotechnology, we embark upon a discourse replete with terminologies as esoteric as they are evocative. This conjunctive nexus heralds a new epoch in healthcare, an era where the infinitesimally small agents of change operate under the aegis of hyper-intelligent

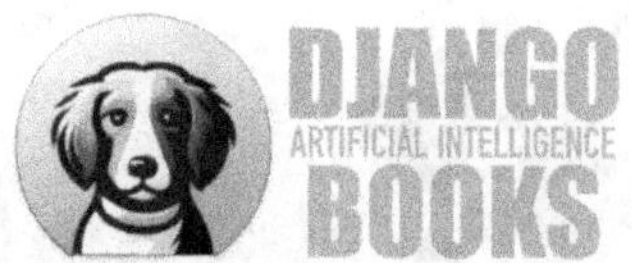

algorithms to engender a paradigm shift in medical interventions and prophylactic strategies.

The premise of integrating AI with nanotechnology in healthcare isn't merely a progressive step; it is a quantum leap towards an envisaged future where therapeutic modalities are not only personalized but are also delivered with precision that parallels the meticulousness of a master horologist crafting a timepiece. Here, AI does not simply direct these nanoscale devices; it imbues them with a semblance of cognitive alacrity, enabling them to make autonomous decisions within the labyrinthine human body.

Consider the intricate ballet of nanobots, those microscopic automatons, deployed into the bloodstream. Under the tutelage of advanced AI, these nanobots could navigate the vascular maze with the agility of a seasoned explorer. They are not aimless wanderers but are equipped with the capabilities to identify and remediate cellular anomalies at their inception. The potential here is not just for treatment but for a revolution in preventative medicine— imagine nanobots that can detect and obliterate cancerous cells before they proliferate, or mend endothelial injuries thus precluding cardiovascular cataclysms.

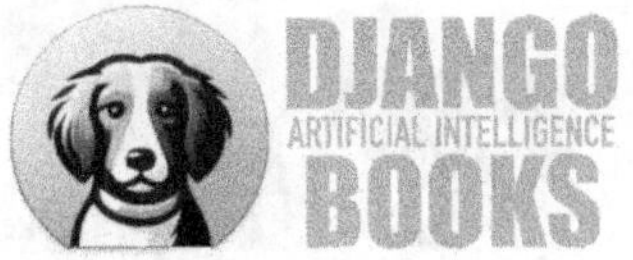

Delving deeper, envisage the synthesis of AI-driven diagnostic nanotechnology. Here, the fusion is so seamless that these nanodevices, circulating discreetly within one's corporeal confines, collect and analyze biological data with an acumen bordering on prescience. This continuous stream of data, when processed through sophisticated AI models, could offer real-time insights into one's health status, preempting diseases with a prescience that verges on the prophetic.

The implications for pharmacology are equally profound. AI could guide the design of nanoscale drug delivery systems that administer medications not just at the requisite site but with a timing so precise, and in dosages so meticulously calibrated, that efficacy is maximized while side effects are all but negated. This level of control is akin to an expert puppeteer who not only commands the strings but anticipates each marionette's next movement.

Furthermore, the convergence of AI with nanotechnology extends its benevolent tendrils into the realm of regenerative medicine. Here, nanotechnology equipped with AI's analytical prowess could orchestrate the repair of tissues and organs at the molecular level. It's a scenario where biological deficits are not merely remedied

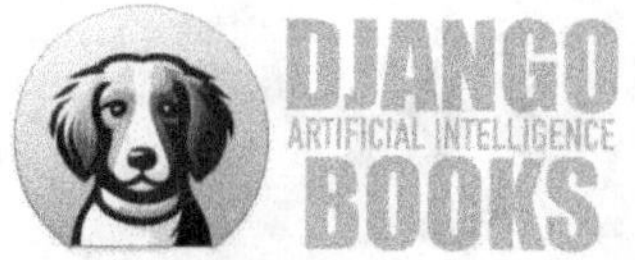

but are preemptively augmented, paving the way for not just healing, but enhanced biological fortitude.

As we prognosticate about this confluence of artificial intelligence and nanotechnology, it becomes clear that we are not merely discussing an incremental enhancement in healthcare. We are contemplating a renaissance in the very methodologies by which human health is maintained and maladies are managed. This is a future where health is not only monitored and maintained continuously by unseen nanoscopic sentinels but is enhanced by interventions so precise that they redefine the very essence of therapeutic precision. Let us then, with both anticipation and a modicum of reverence for the technological wizardry at our disposal, look forward to a future where health is not a mere absence of disease, but a dynamically maintained state of optimal well-being.

As we ascend the vertiginous slopes of technological advancement, where artificial intelligence melds with the very sinews of healthcare, the imperative to lace our boots with the sturdy straps of ethics and governance cannot be overstated. Indeed, navigating this terrain requires a blend of philosophical acumen and practical sagacity, much like trying to solve a Rubik's Cube while riding a unicycle—

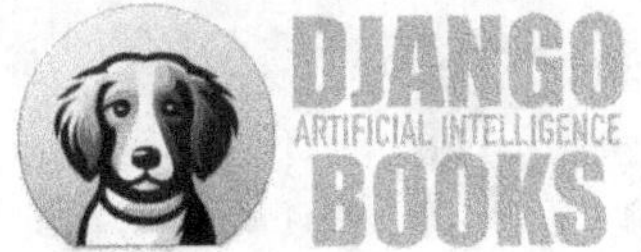

challenging, but undeniably exhilarating and profoundly essential.

In this futuristic tableau, where AI not only diagnoses but potentially dictates our health choices, the question of ethics looms as large as a billboard in Times Square. Imagine, if you will, an AI so advanced that it suggests not just when you might take a brisk walk but also whom you might consider dating based on genetic compatibility and psychological profiling. Intrusive? Possibly. Useful? Perhaps. Ethical? Well... depends on how well the date went! ;)

This scenario beckons us to the colossal task of drafting what could only be described as a 'Magna Carta' for the AI health governance realm. This isn't your typical bureaucratic red tape or your run-of-the-mill legislative snooze-fest. No, this is about crafting guidelines with the precision of a Swiss watchmaker and the foresight of a seasoned chess grandmaster, ensuring that AI in health acts not as a domineering overlord but as a benevolent aide steeped in the sacrosanct principles of do no harm, fairness, and autonomy.

Imagine ethical guidelines that ensure AI respects your personal data like a squirrel treasures its nuts—guarded

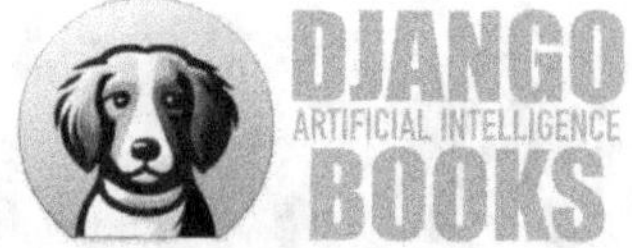

under lock and key, only to be revealed in the direst of needs and under the strictest confidentiality. These guidelines must be robust, yet flexible; prescriptive, yet permissive enough to foster innovation without letting the proverbial genie out of the bottle to wreak havoc.

Moreover, as we plunge headfirst into this brave new world, the governance of such AI systems will need to be as dynamic as the technology itself. Static rules won't do. We need live, breathing policies that evolve as swiftly as the algorithms they seek to regulate. This means establishing oversight bodies with the agility of Olympic gymnasts, capable of somersaulting through rapidly changing technological landscapes while keeping their eyes firmly on the ethical gold medal.

One might also consider the establishment of a global consortium, akin to the United Nations of AI Health Governance—let's call it the "Health AI Harmony and Ethics Society" (HAHES), tasked not only with keeping AI's immense capabilities in check but also with promoting its most altruistic applications. This body would not merely police but would provide a platform for sharing best practices, a symposium of sorts, where the brightest minds

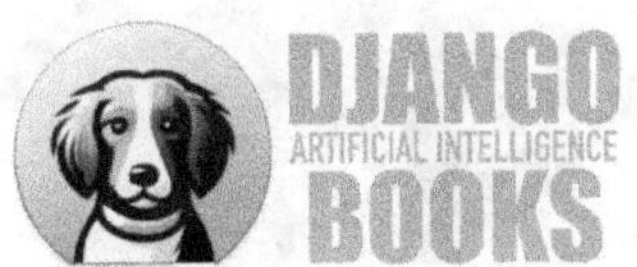

congregate not to compete but to collaborate, ensuring AI is leveraged for the collective boon of global health.

And let us not eschew the humorous side of things. Envision AI designed to maintain not only physical health but also mental well-being through doses of humor, administered as needed, to keep spirits buoyant. After all, laughter could very well be the best medicine, especially when prescribed by an AI with impeccable comedic timing.

In sum, as we march toward this future, rich with potential yet fraught with pitfalls, let us do so with a vigilant eye on the ethical compass, ensuring that as we harness the formidable powers of AI to heal, enhance, and extend human lives, we remain steadfast in our commitment to uphold dignity, autonomy, and fairness. For in this grand journey of health innovation, it is not merely the destination that matters but also the integrity of the path we tread.

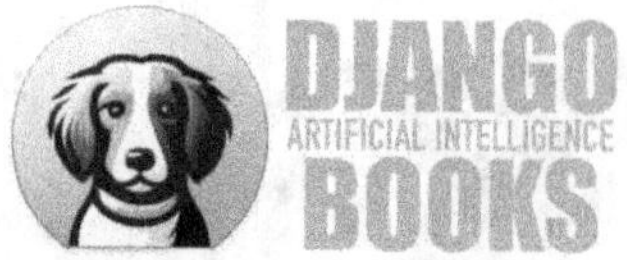

Conclusion

As we prepare to close the cover on this compendious compendium of futuristic foresights and practical prescriptions, let us not simply walk away with a head full of knowledge but stride forward with a veritable blueprint for actionable change. The convergence of artificial intelligence with the multifaceted world of healthcare promises not only to recalibrate our current paradigms of wellness but also to redefine what it means to live a healthy, fulfilled life.

In our journey through the chapters, from the nascent genesis of AI in healthcare, weaving through the sophisticated labyrinths of mental health, personalized medicine, and the zenith of ethical AI governance, we've unearthed a treasure trove of insights. These are not mere theoretical musings but actionable, tangible strategies designed to elevate your existence. Each page of this tome was crafted not as a panegyric to the potential of technology but as a pragmatic guide to harnessing this potential for personal health enhancement.

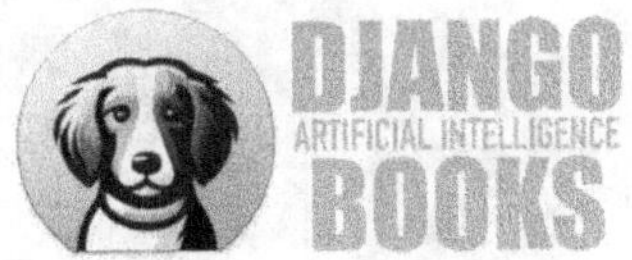

This volume was scribed with the hope that readers would not just passively absorb information but actively engage with it, employing AI as both a scalpel and a scaffold in the architecture of their health regimen. Whether it was through understanding the subtle intricacies of AI-powered wearables that monitor every pulse and palpitation, or through exploring the avant-garde realms where AI and quantum computing amalgamate to fabricate medical marvels, this book aimed to provide you with the knowledge to be not just a bystander but a proactive architect of your health destiny.

Moreover, as we contemplated the ethical dimensions and the future governance of AI in health, it was not out of a desire to stoke fears but to ignite a beacon of stewardship, ensuring that as we advance into this brave new world, we do so with our moral compasses steadfastly oriented towards equity, empathy, and excellence. The discourse on ethics and governance serves as a clarion call to all stakeholders in the health AI ecosystem to wield this powerful tool with wisdom and circumspection.

The horizon of health, augmented by artificial intelligence, stretches vast and inviting before us. It beckons not with the cold glow of screens and the sterile

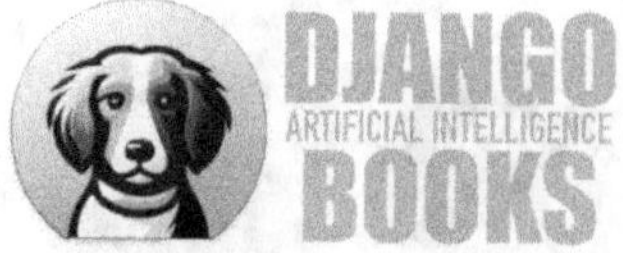

beep of machines but with the warm promise of enhanced longevity, diminished disease, and an unprecedented understanding of the human body and mind. As this book concludes, let it mark not the end of your quest for knowledge but the beginning of an enlightened, AI-infused approach to personal health.

Let each reader take from this tome not just ideas but inspiration—not merely plans but a passion—to employ AI in forging a future where health is not a fleeting state but a perpetual, dynamic journey. With AI as your steadfast companion, navigate this journey with the judiciousness of a sage and the joy of a soul untethered from the apprehensions of ailment.

Thus, as we bid adieu to this textual journey, remember that the true voyage lies ahead. It is yours to chart with care, courage, and a copious dose of curiosity. Embrace AI, but steer it with the hands of a seasoned helmsman, knowing well that the seas of technology are vast, but the potential for health and happiness is vaster still. Here's to your health, enhanced not just by artificial intelligence but by an authentically invigorated spirit of human ingenuity and innovation.

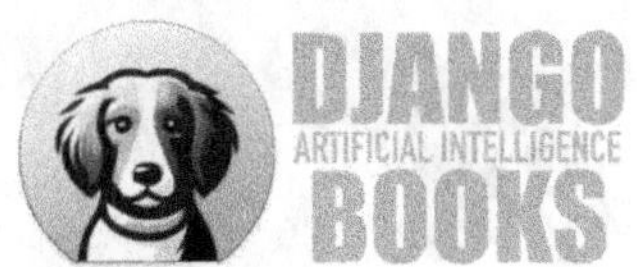

Please Leave a Review

Hey there, savvy reader! If this book is helping you enhance your health with a dash of AI magic, why not take a moment to sprinkle some karma into the universe? Your review could be just what future readers need to discover this gem. It doesn't have to be a novel—just a few seconds for a few words will do!

Simply click the link or point your phone at the QR code. Thanks in advance for sharing your thoughts—trust me, your good health karma is about to skyrocket!!

Click Here to Leave Review

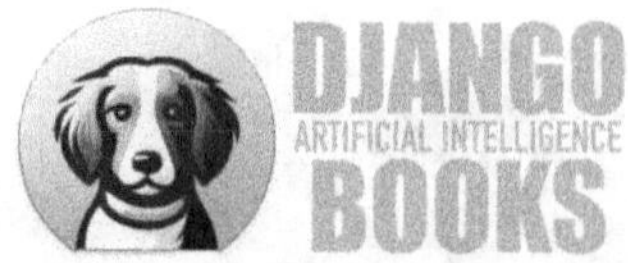

All Django AI Books (With Great Discounts)

Did you like this book?

Well, there are many more!

Check them all out and get GREAT DISCOUNTS

by clicking this link:

https://djangoartificialintelligencebooks.typedream.app

OR

by pointing your phone camera to this QR code:

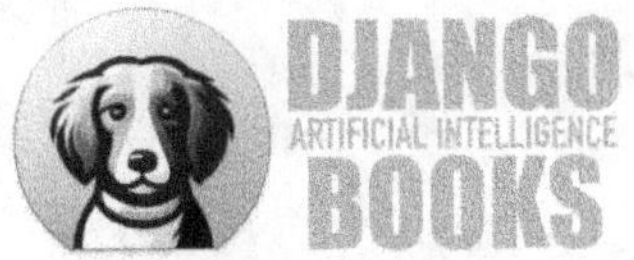